A Colour Atlas of

Diseases of the Domestic Fowl & Turkey

C.J. Randall

MA VetMB MRCVS

Ministry of Agriculture, Fisheries and Food
Veterinary Laboratory,
Eskgrove, Lasswade,
Midlothian,
Scotland.

Wolfe Medical Publications Ltd

© Crown copyright 1985
Published by permission of the
Controller of Her Majesty's Stationery Office
Published by Wolfe Medical Publications Ltd 1985
Reprinted 1986
Printed by W. S.Cowell Ltd, 8 Buttermarket, Ipswich,
England
ISBN 0 7234 0827 0
For a full list of Wolfe Veterinary Colour Atlases, plus
forthcoming titles, please write to Wolfe Medical
Publications Ltd, Wolfe House, 3 Conway Street, London
W1P 6HE

Contents

Acknowledgements

I am very grateful to both past and present colleagues for discussions about many aspects of poultry disease. In particular I thank J F Harbourne, C T McCrea, A R Hunter, J W Macdonald and Helen G R Jones. Much useful advice on the draft manuscript was given by Mr J W Macdonald, Lasswade Laboratory, Dr M Pattison, Sun Valley Poultry Ltd, Dr L N Payne, Houghton Poultry Research Station, and Drs W G Siller and P A L Wight, Agricultural Research Council, Poultry Research Centre. I am most grateful for their help. Dr J G Ross, Director, Lasswade Laboratory, is thanked for giving continuous support and sympathetic encouragement throughout.

I am indebted to the following for providing me with valuable transparencies: the late Dr J E Wilson, previously Director of the Lasswade Laboratory, for **63-67**, **96**, **138**, **149**, **176**, **191** and **247**, Dr R C Jones, Sub-Department of Avian Medicine, University of Liverpool, for **120-123** (copyright for these four pictures rests with Dr R C Jones), and to Mr D E Gray, Librarian at the Central Veterinary Laboratory, for arranging the loan of **48**, **68-70**, **85**, **98**, **99**, **102** and **103** from the Library's collection. I also thank Mr Gray for undertaking the task of preparing the Index. Sections of reticuloendotheliosis virus-induced tumours in turkeys and round heart in the fowl were kindly provided, respectively, by Dr J S McDougall, Houghton Poultry Research Station and by Dr C Riddell, Western College of Veterinary Medicine, University of Saskatchewan.

The tissue sections photographed were prepared by the staff of the Pathology section at Lasswade who are thanked for dealing expertly with many requests. Mr W Gordon, ably assisted by Mr S Lees, Miss S M Clark and Mrs E Melvin, helped at all stages with the photography. I am indebted to them for their enthusiasm and skill. Mrs L Johnstone is thanked for cheerfully typing the text.

Preface

The purpose of this atlas is to provide the diagnostician with photographs of the main post-mortem and histopathological features of common diseases in the domestic fowl and turkey. The atlas does not aim to cover the other procedures that may be required to confirm a diagnosis. The text has been kept to a minimum and is intended to be read in conjunction with textbooks of poultry disease (see page 111).

Selection of conditions reflects the author's experience in Great Britain. Inevitably this has led to the omission of some diseases of interest but photographs of less frequently seen disorders are included where they have been thought appropriate. In the main, the photographs have been assembled during the last ten years; diagnostically they span a period of seventeen years.

Diseases that might be usefully considered together are arranged under main group headings rather than being listed alphabetically. A miscellaneous group of conditions, whose aetiologies are generally understood, is listed separately from those of uncertain or unknown cause. Names have been selected for some conditions (**236-246**) that are seen as distinct entities but which still require further definition.

All photomicrographs are of tissue sections stained with haematoxylin and eosin unless stated otherwise. In two instances sections from species other than the fowl and turkey are shown. Water soluble acrylic resins have been used occasionally for tissue embedding to show particular features and this use is also indicated in the legends. Magnifications of photomicrographs have been omitted as these were thought to be of doubtful value.

Bacterial Diseases

Coli bacillosis
(including peritonitis in layers and salpingitis)

1 Coli septicaemia. *Escherichia coli* causing severe pericarditis, perihepatitis and air sacculitis in a broiler following a primary viral infection of the respiratory tract. The fibrinous exudate covering one lobe of the liver has been cut to show the surface of the organ beneath. Hepatic and pericardial lesions of this type are occasionally seen in some systemic salmonella infections in young chickens and turkeys (*see* **59**).

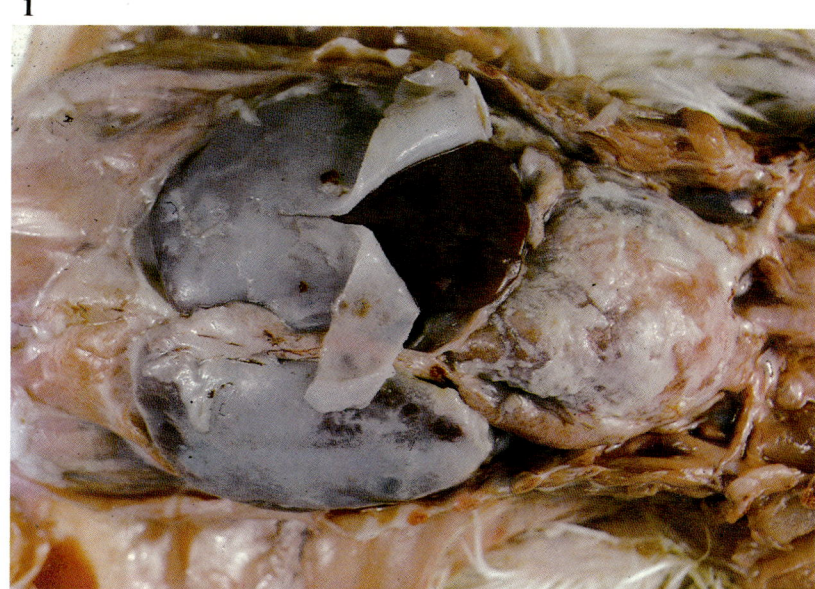

2 Coli septicaemia. Liver section showing the fibrinous nature of the deposit on the surface of the organ. Martius scarlet blue.

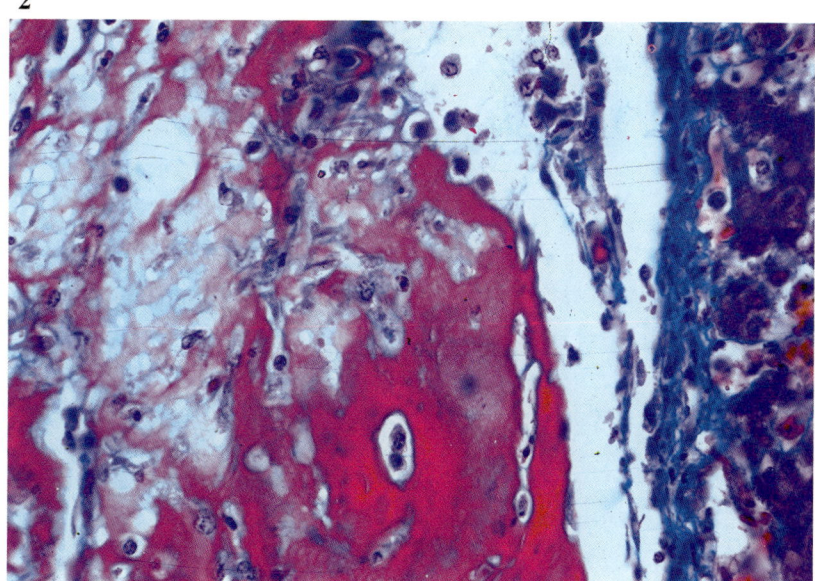

3 Coli septicaemia. Eosinophilic coagulum in a periarteriolar sheath in the spleen. This feature is frequently encountered in cases of Coli septicaemia. It is usually marked in this infection but similar changes may occur in other septicaemias and viraemias.

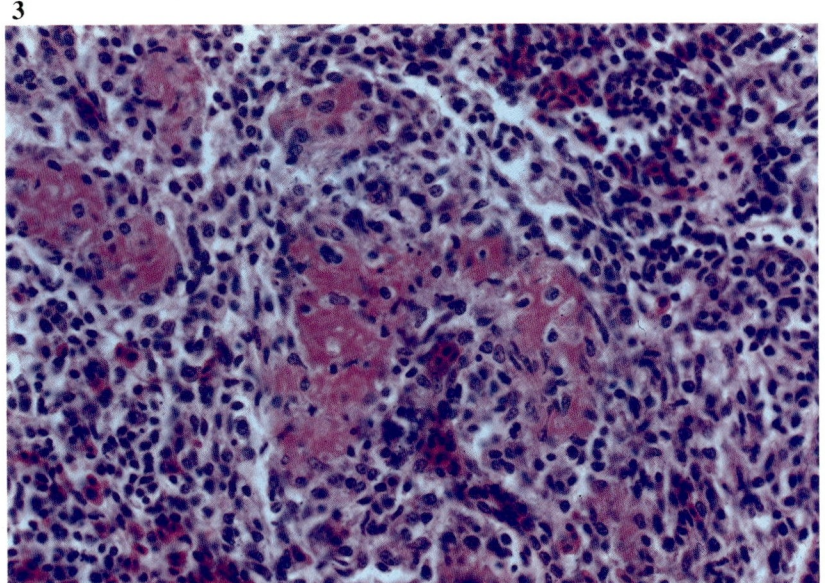

4 Coli septicaemia. Synovitis of hock joints is commonly found in broilers. Creamish coloured exudate tends to be tinged with brown. There may be concurrent lesions of osteomyelitis, particularly at the proximal tibiotarsal growth plate (*see* **31**).

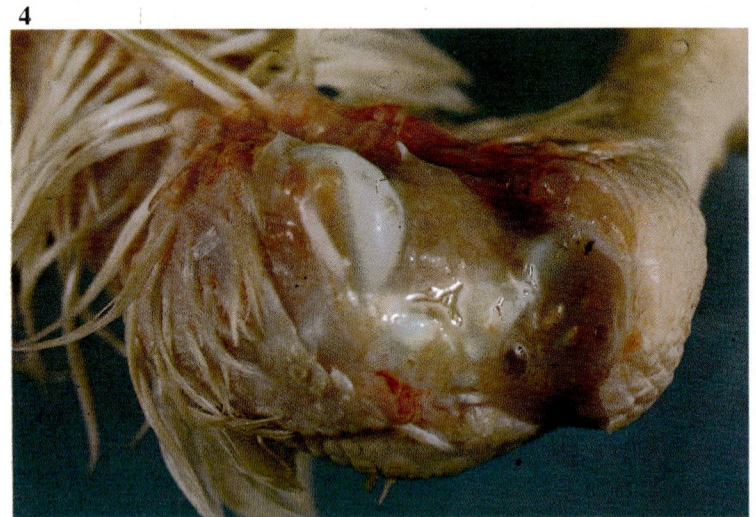

5 Coli septicaemia. Salpingitis in a 3-week-old broiler. Inflammation of the immature oviduct is a relatively common finding in broilers.

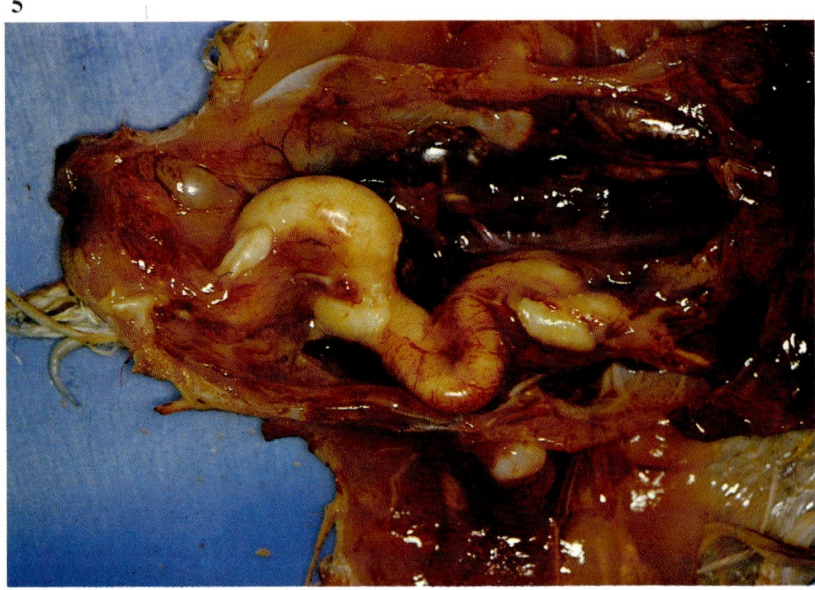

6 Coli septicaemia. Turkey grower. Lesions were confined in this instance to an overall carcase congestion and a marked congestion of the spleen (arrow). This bird gave a serologically positive reaction for *Mycoplasma meleagridis* antibodies. In this species pericarditis may accompany Coli septicaemia but fibrinous deposits on the liver are less common. Greening of the liver may take place after exposure to the air.

6

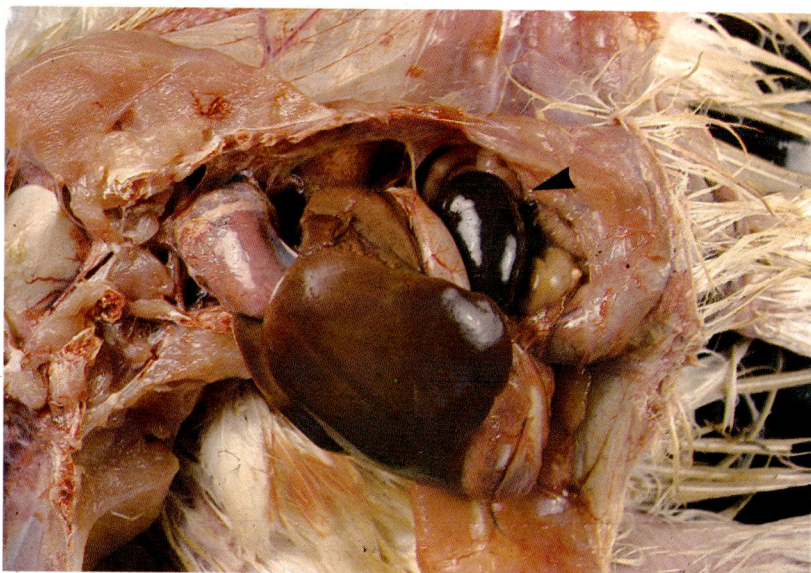

7 *E. coli* is isolated from the great majority of cases of peritonitis in adult laying fowl. The condition is often termed 'egg peritonitis', but the presence of yolk mixed with the exudate is variable. Birds dying in acute stages are usually septicaemic.

7

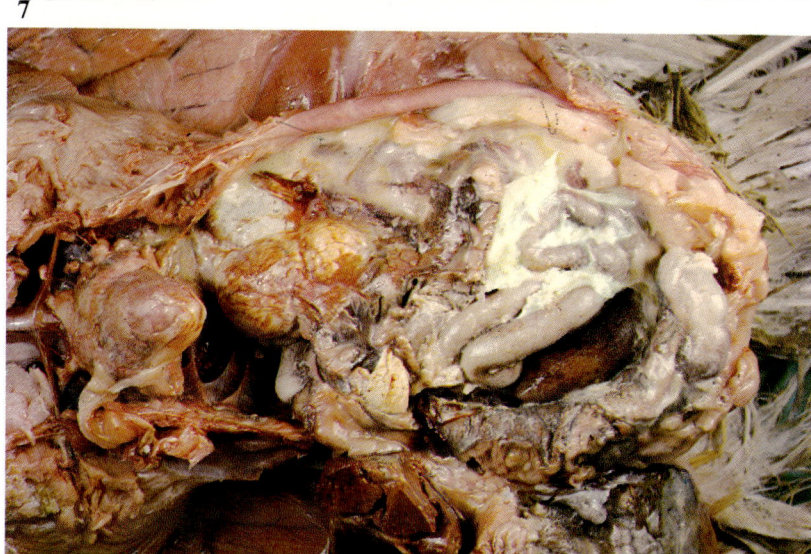

8 Laying fowl may die as a result of acute salpingitis. Many survive this episode, with the result that the inflammatory exudate becomes partially organised. The affected oviducts may be extremely enlarged and occupy most of the abdominal cavity. *E. coli* is usually isolated from these lesions.

8

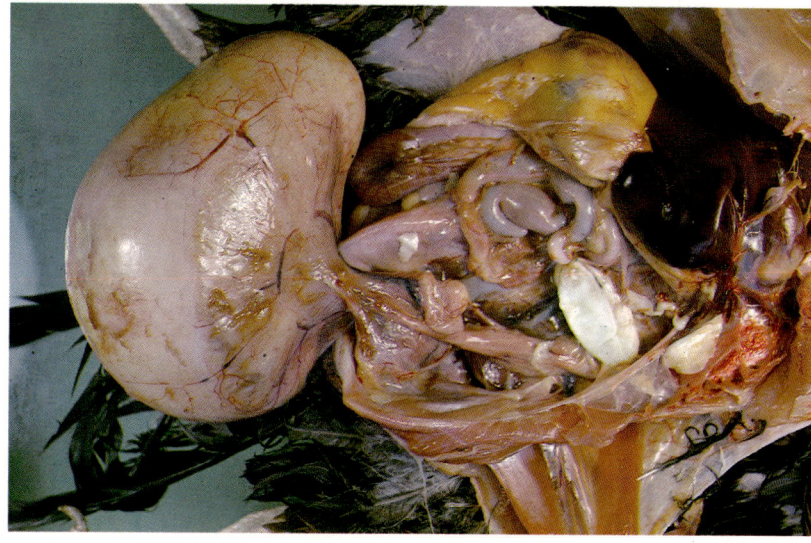

9 The exudate contained within the oviduct of **8** has been cut to show the onion-layered texture of the inflammatory exudate and, in this case, a shelled egg.

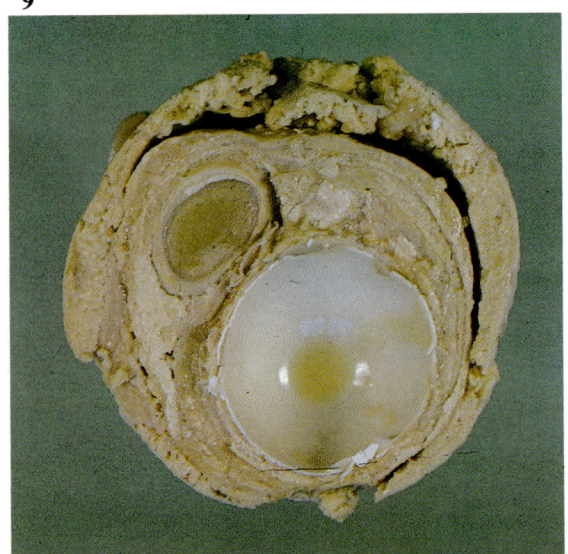

10 Layering of fibrinous exudate within an oviduct. Martius scarlet blue.

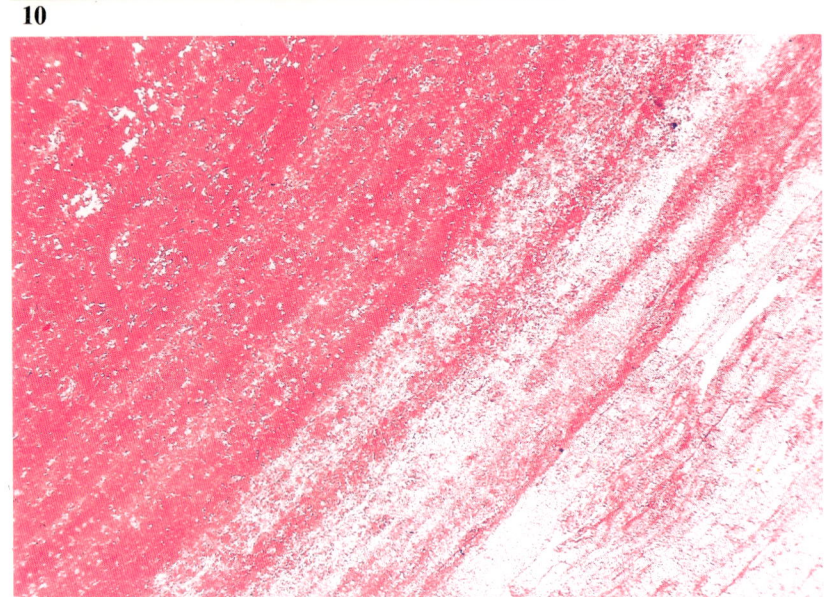

11 Coli granuloma (Hjärres disease) affecting the caeca of a laying fowl. The lesions must be distinguished from those of tuberculosis, which is best done histologically (*see* **53**).

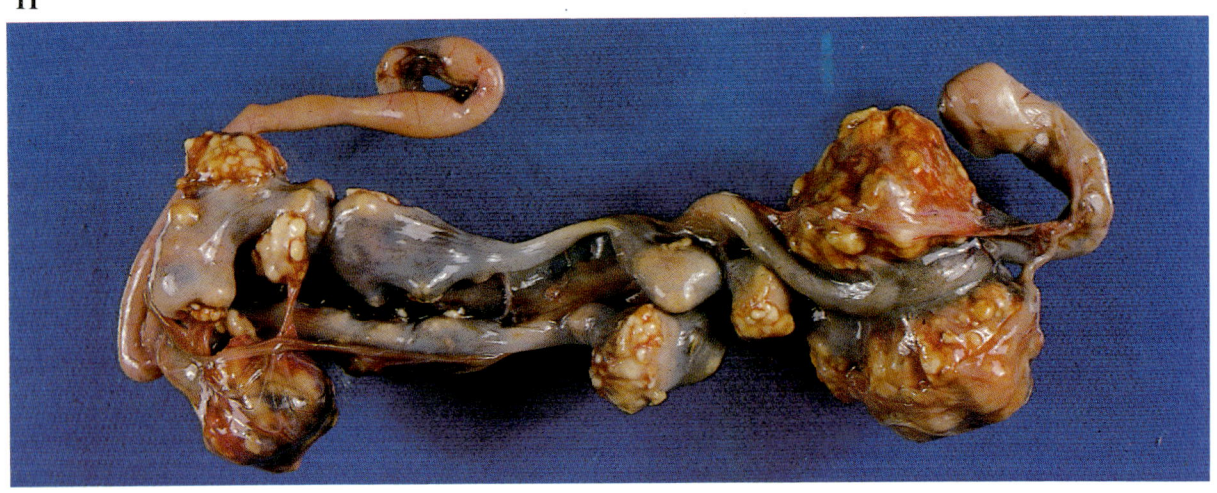

12 Coli granuloma. Cross section of a granuloma from **11**.

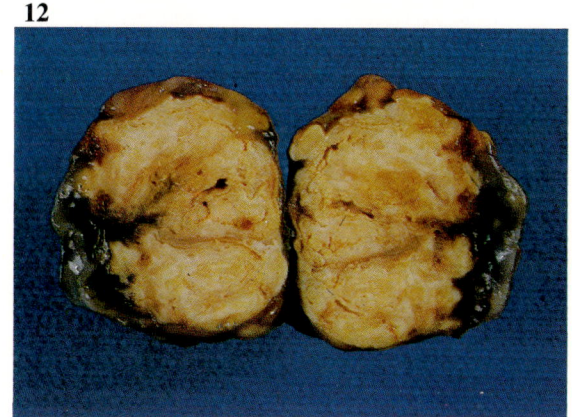

Fowl cholera *(Pasteurella multocida)*

13 Swollen wattles in a male broiler breeder due to *P. multocida* infection. The affected males may be slightly depressed in localised infection of this type. Swollen wattles may also occur amongst the females, as well as a cellulitis, which is usually seen over the head and neck.

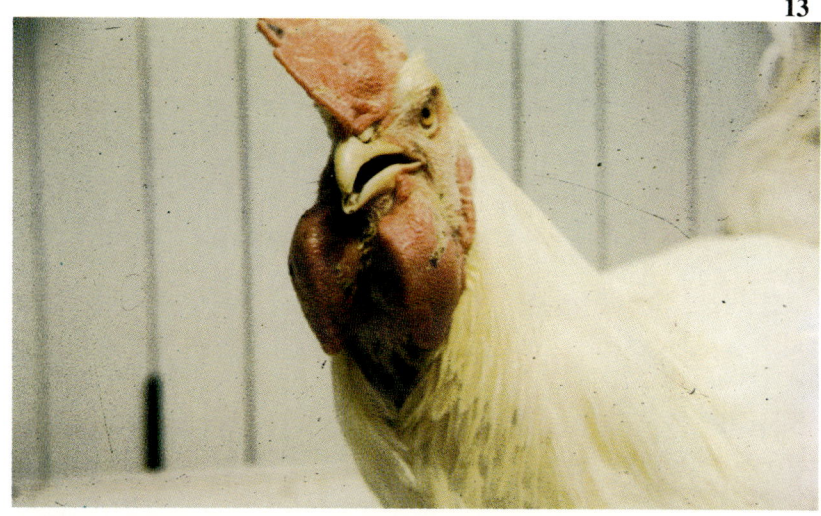

14 Core of pus in a swollen wattle of a broiler breeder hen. *P. multocida* can be isolated from most acute lesions of this type but only rarely from chronic abscesses. This may give rise to some diagnostic difficulty as wattle abscesses can be caused by a variety of bacteria.

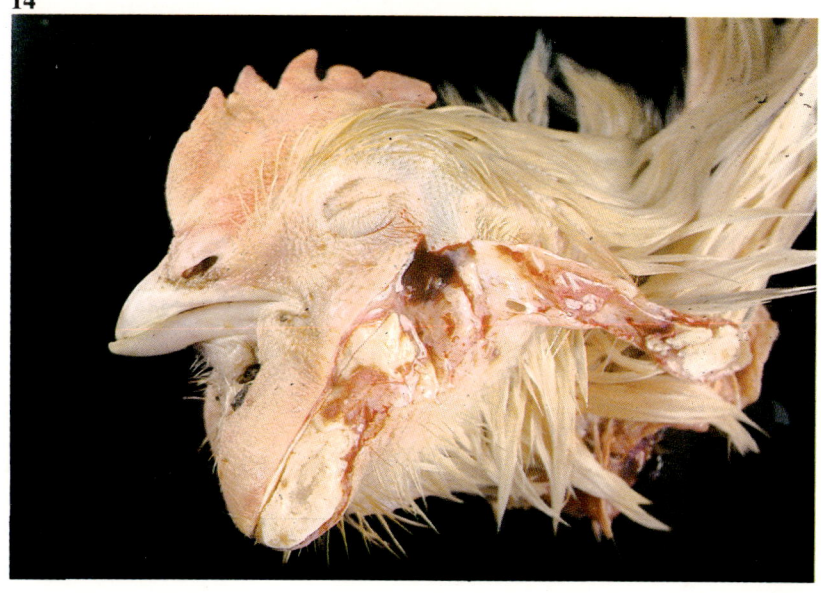

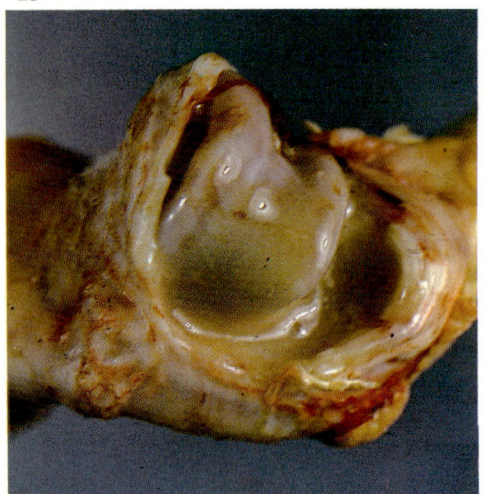

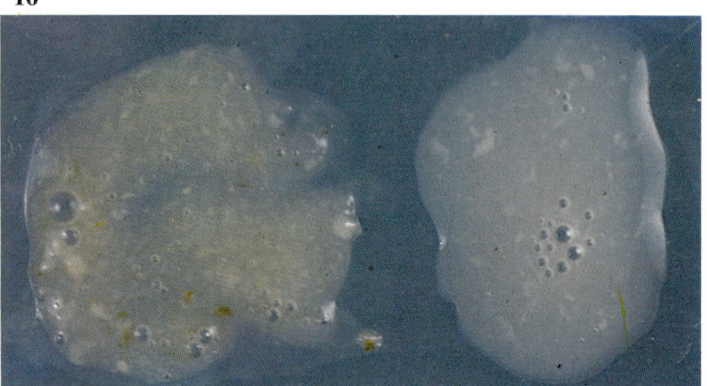

15 Purulent synovitis in a hock joint of an adult broiler breeder cockerel. Lameness may be a presenting clinical sign in some outbreaks.

16 Comparison of pale flecked exudate (right) from a case of staphyloccal synovitis with the more yellow-tinged granular exudate obtained from a *P. multocida* infected joint.

17 Peritonitis is often found in adult layers in septicaemic forms of the infection.

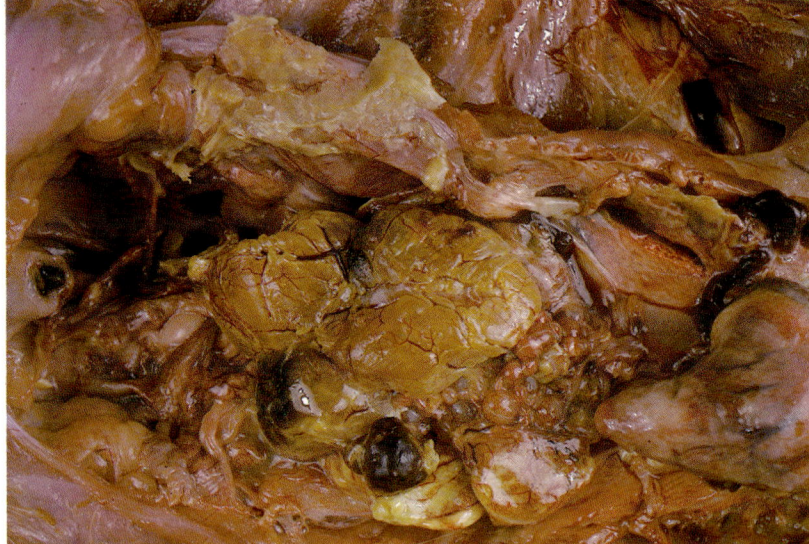

18 Blood stained mucus in the mouth of a septicaemic turkey breeder.

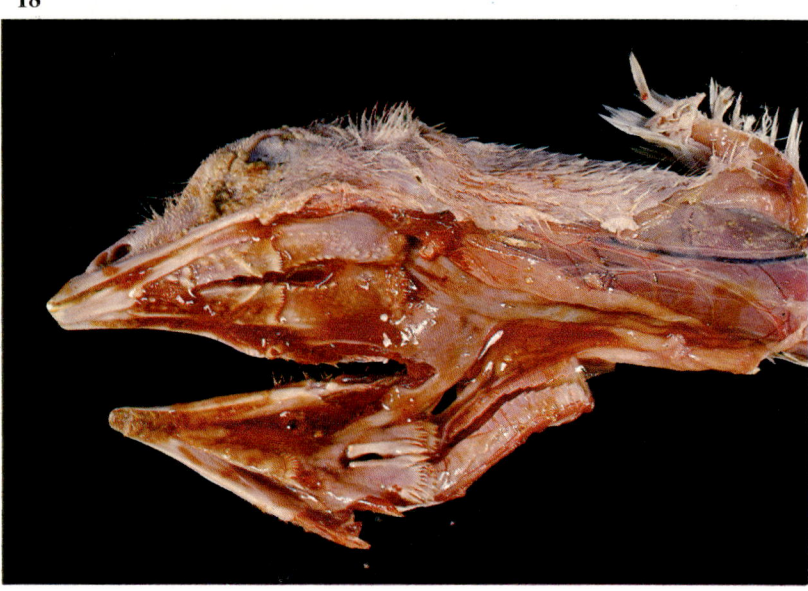

19 Purulent pleuropneumonia in a
10-week-old turkey grower. This bird
was unvaccinated. Pneumonic lesions are more commonly seen in the
turkey than in the fowl.

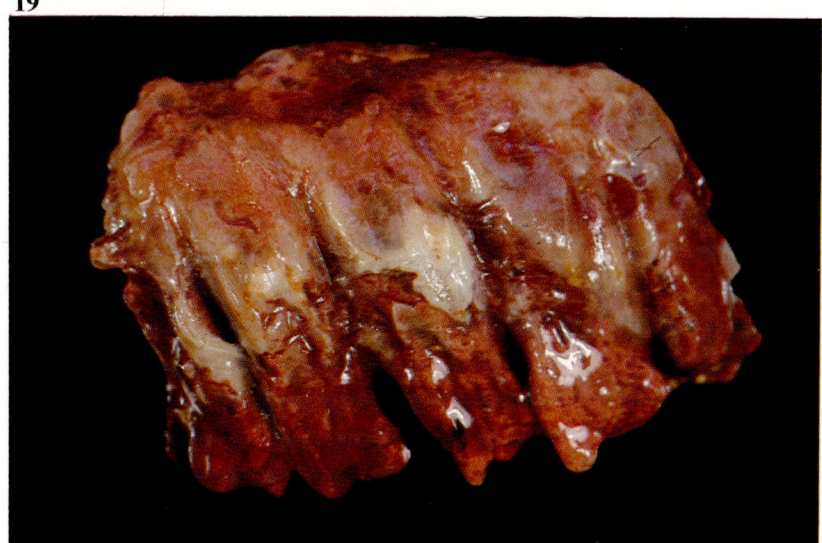

20 Masses of pasteurellas within a
lung of a turkey that died from a dual
infection of *P. multocida* and Newcastle disease.

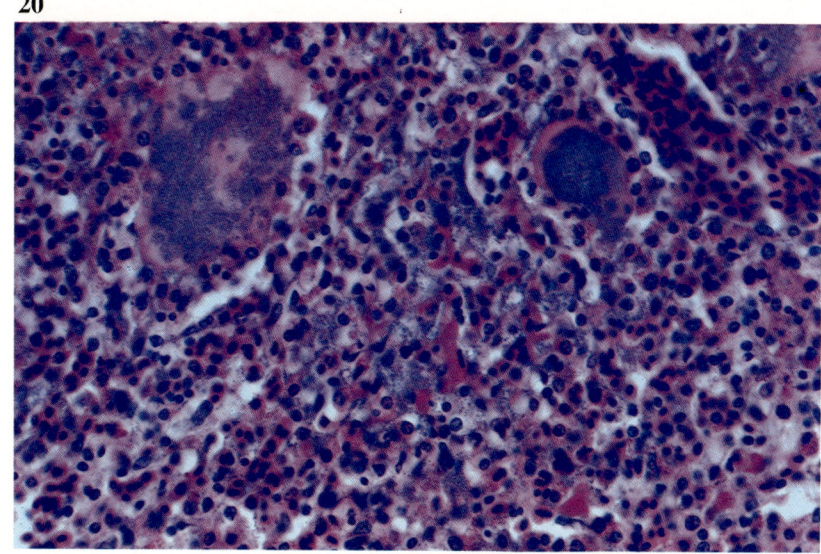

21 Acute pneumonia in a 22-week-
old broiler breeder. Pasteurellas
usually stain more basophilically
(arrow) in H & E preparations than
most other commonly encountered
Gram-negative organisms. The tissue
to the right of the bacteria is necrotic,
that to the left is reactive.

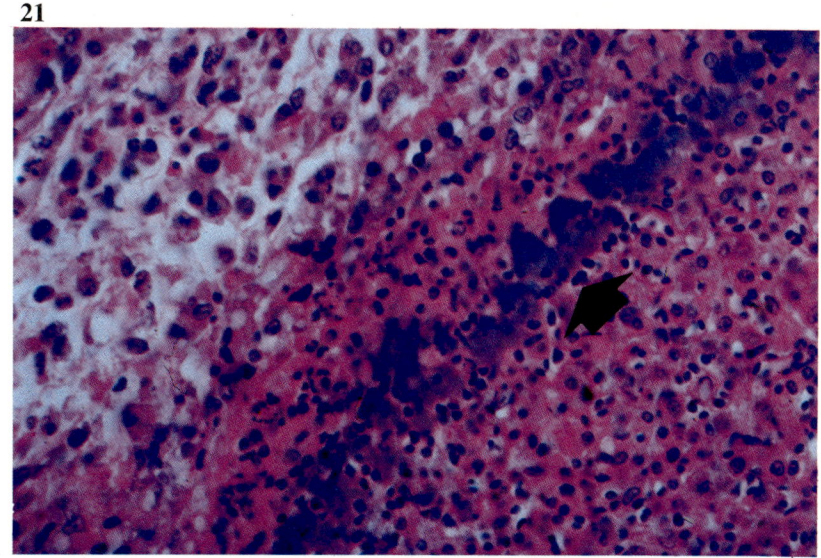

Yolk sac infection and omphalitis

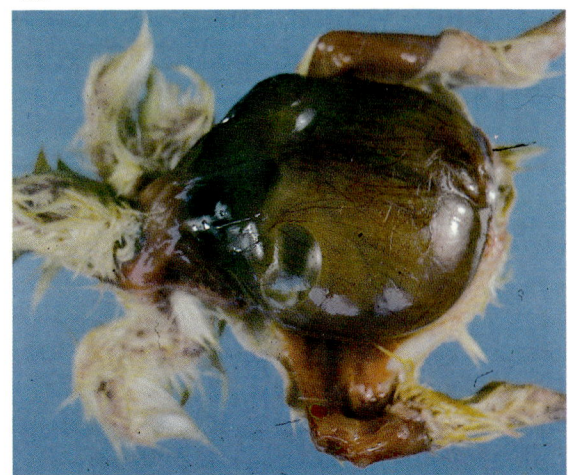

22 The abdomen of this chick is greatly distended as a result of yolk sac infection. Most birds die at 3-4 days of age. There may be an accompanying omphalitis. The carcasses often smell unpleasantly.

23 Intense inflammation of an infected yolk sac.

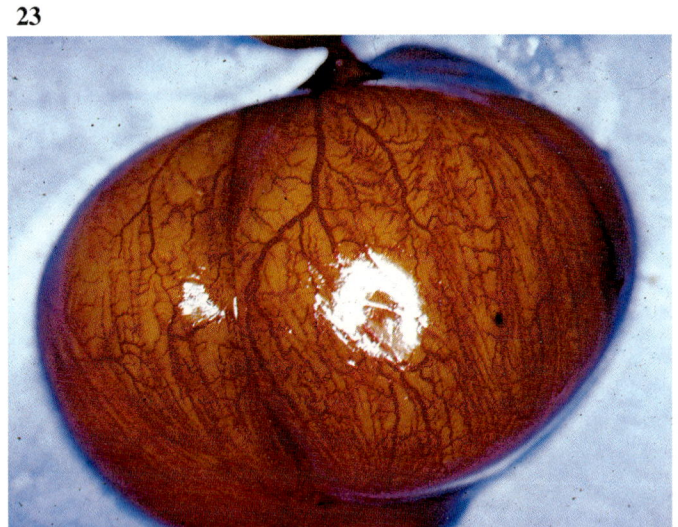

24 The normal consistency of the yolk is lost and in the acute stages of the disease the contents are thin and have a strong odour. The presence of soft and friable viscera together with moist abdominal skin and down led to the condition being called "mushy chick disease".

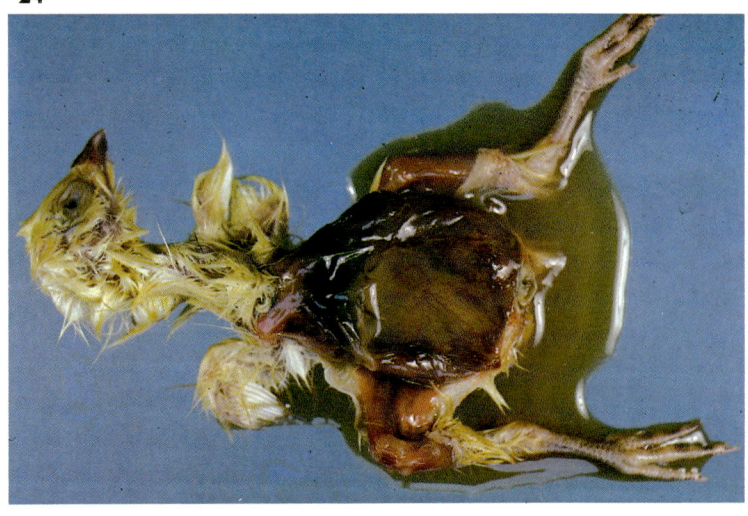

25 The contents of the infected yolk sac may become inspissated if the chick or poult survives into the second week of life. Infected yolk sac remnants containing deeply pigmented cheesy material are a frequent incidental post-mortem finding in older birds.

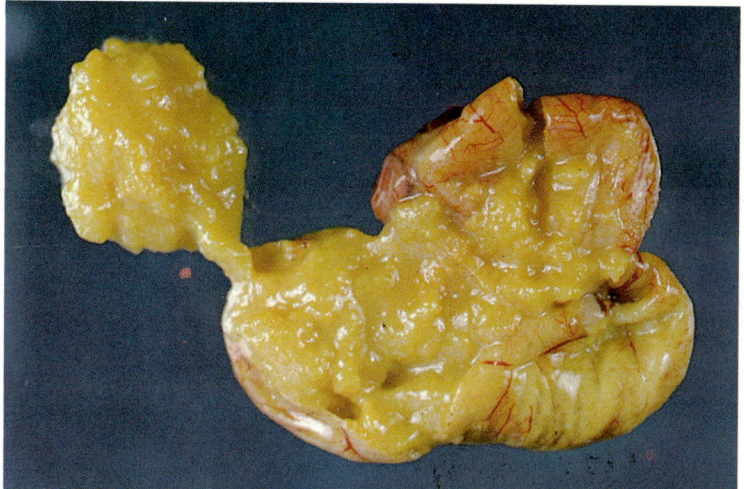
25

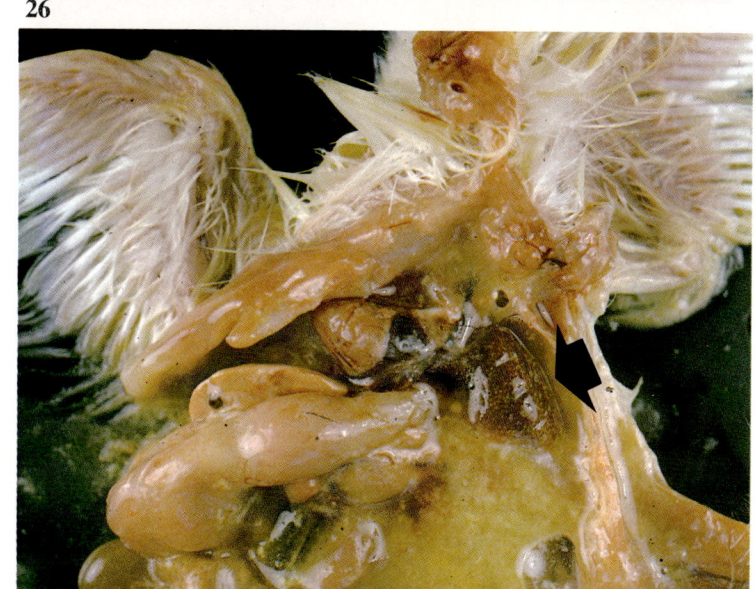
26

26 Intense lung congestion (arrow) occurs in the acute stages. Note the pool of yolky material within the abdominal cavity.

27 A wide variety of bacteria may be isolated either in single or mixed infections. *E. coli* is frequently cultured from affected birds and may lead to classical lesions of Coli septicaemia (*see* **1**) towards the end of the first week. Synovitis and osteomyelitis can also be seen in coliform and other infections introduced by this route.

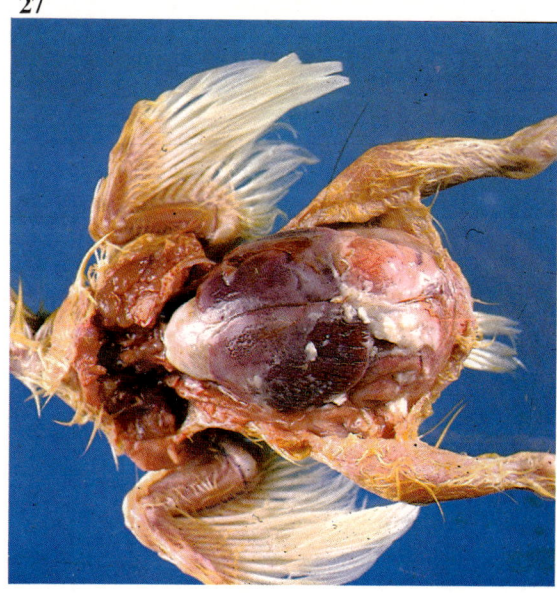
27

Staphylococcal infection *(Staphylococcus aureus)*

28 Synovitis associated with staphyloccocal infection in a 10-week-old broiler breeder. This infection is most often seen during the rearing period. The base of the gastrocnemius tendon is usually swollen as well as the joint. Reoviruses may need to be considered as primary infecting agents in some outbreaks (*see* **120-123**).

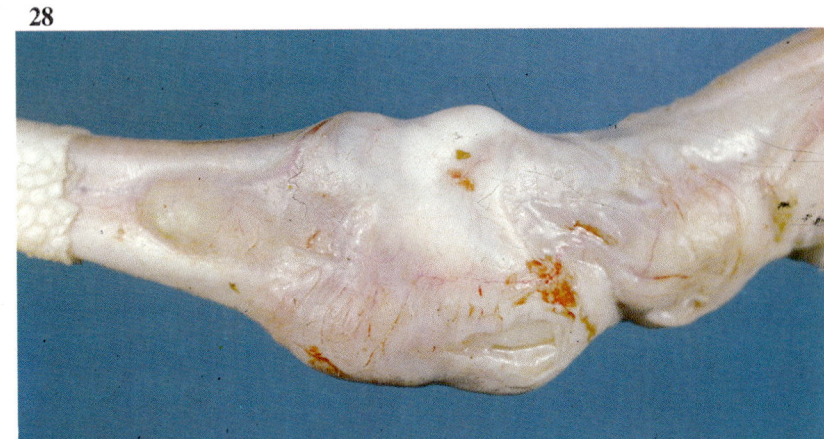

29 The hock joint in **28** has been opened to show the large quantity of purulent exudate. This lesion often extends into the sheaths of the digital flexor tendons and the gastrocnemius tendon.

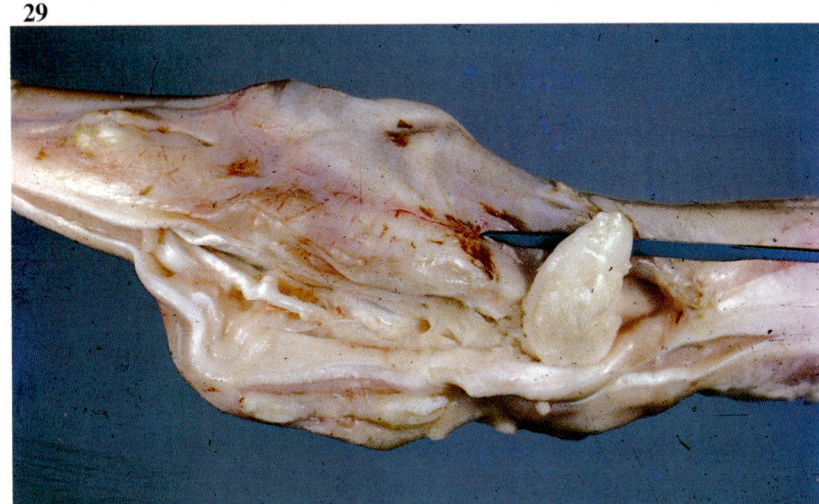

30 Chronic case of staphylococcal arthritis in a young broiler breeder showing erosion of the cartilage over the distal tibiotarsal condyles.

31 Osteomyelitis in a turkey grower. The infected tissue is pale and crumbly and situated distal to the proximal growth plate of the tibiotarsus. Osteomyelitis is frequently found at this site in broiler types and turkey growers. Staphylococci (and *E. coli*) are often isolated from such lesions. The long bones – particularly the tibiotarsus – should always be split when young birds are presented with a history of lameness.

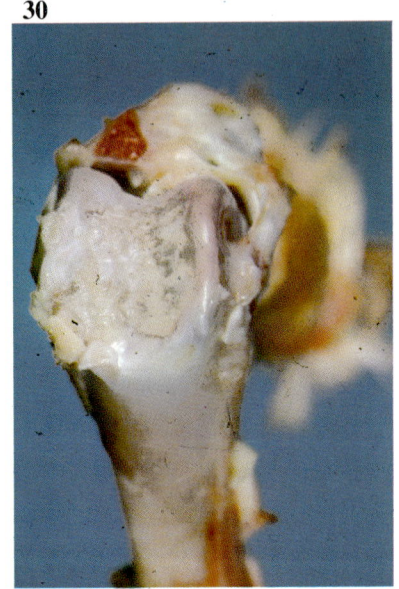

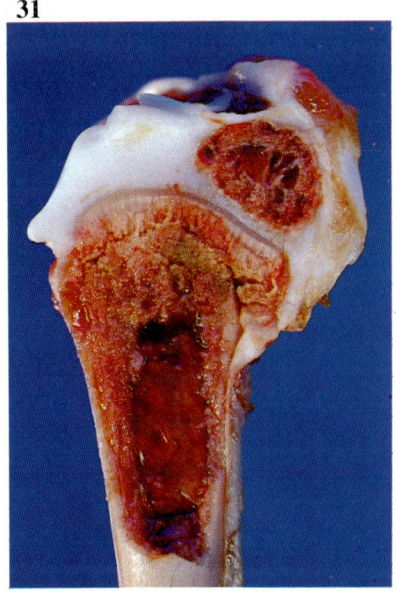

32 Osteomyelitis. A small in-flammatory focus in a tibiotarsal growth plate containing numerous clusters of bacteria.

32

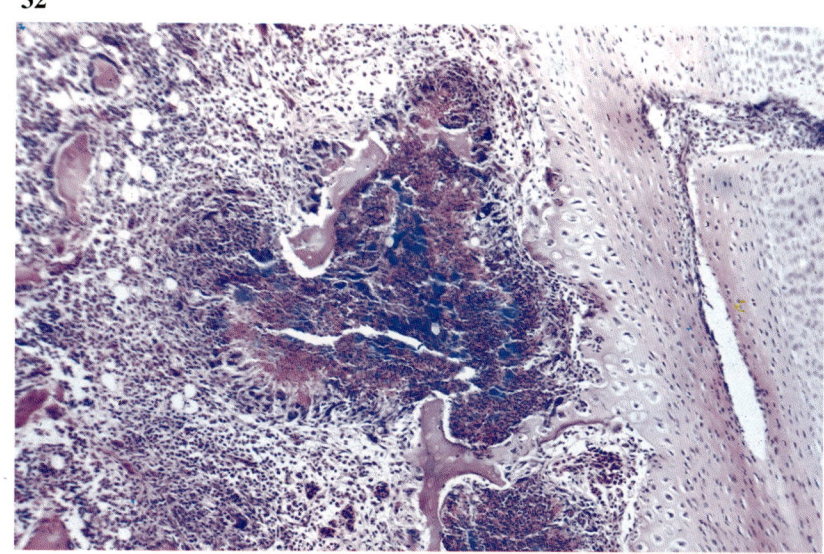

33 Clearly defined necrotic lesions in the liver of a 15-week-old turkey breeder that had been de-beaked 10 days previously. There were concurrent lesions of synovitis. Hepatic lesions of this type are commonly seen in laying fowl in association with vegetative endocarditis. Staphylococcal septicaemias occur from time to time in commercial and breeding hens with few lesions other than generalised carcase and hepatic congestion.

33

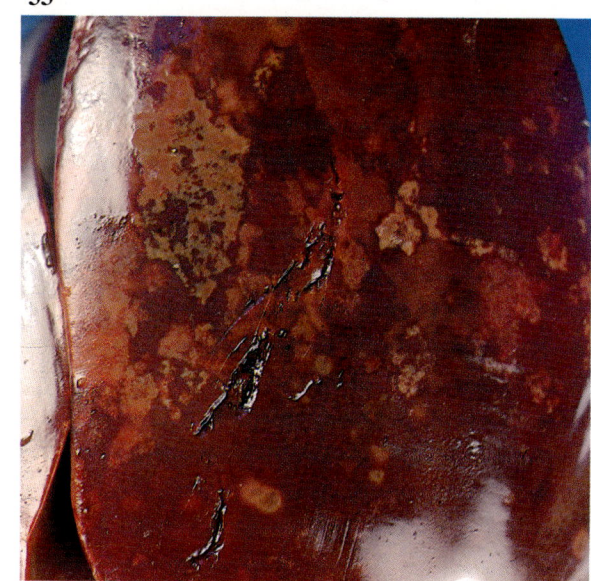

34 Liver lesions similar to those in **33** often show a few scattered colonies of Gram-positive cocci surrounded by large zones of necrosis and with little inflammatory reaction at the periphery. Gram.

34

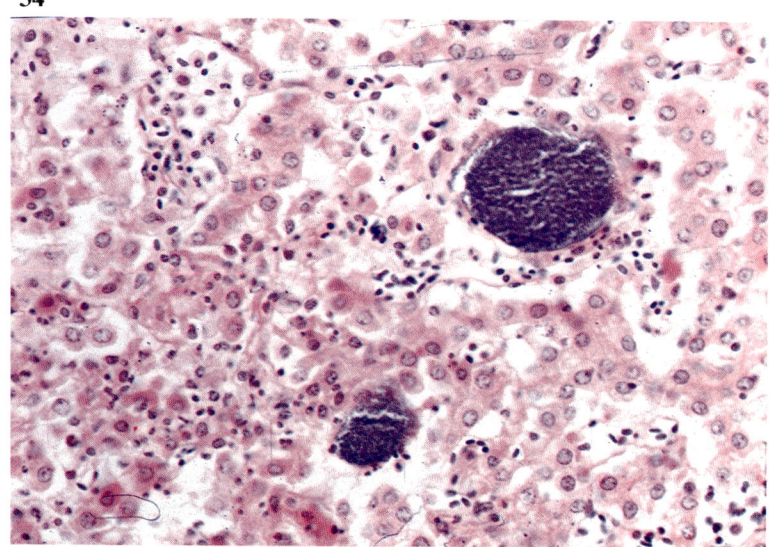

35 Sporadic deaths, particularly in commercial layers, are often caused by vegetative endocarditis of the left atrio-ventricular valve. Streptococci may also be isolated from vegetative lesions of this type.

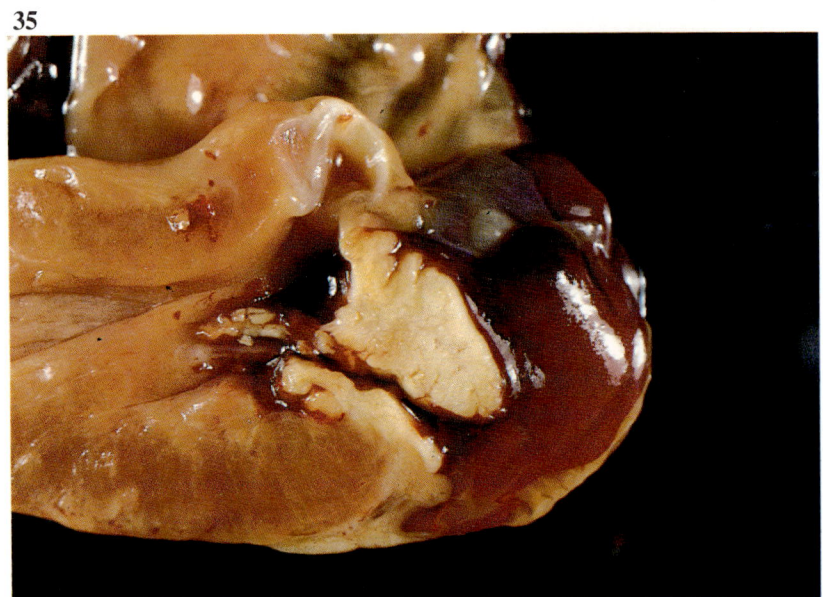

Necrotic enteritis

36 Early necrotic enteritis in the small intestine of a 3-week-old broiler. The mucosal surface is abnormally pale due to necrosis of the tips of the villi.

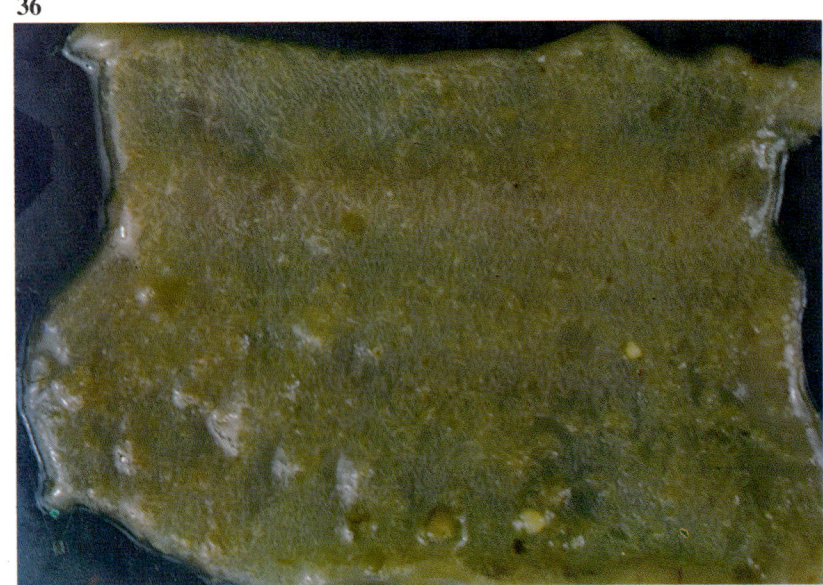

37 Advanced lesion. The necrotic mucous membrane is fissured and detaching from the deeper layers. Sloughing of parts of the mucous membrane may give the serous surface a faintly speckled appearance. Most of the upper small intestine is usually involved in the lesion. The condition is seen predominantly in young broilers and broiler breeders (*see* **189**).

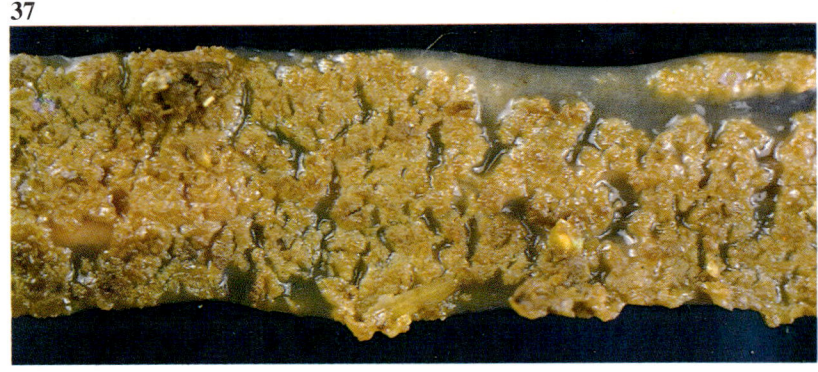

38 Smear of small intestinal contents showing the predominance of Gram-positive bacilli. These organisms are often decaying and stain variably. Profuse growths of *Clostridium perfringens* are isolated from intestines of birds that have died. Gram.

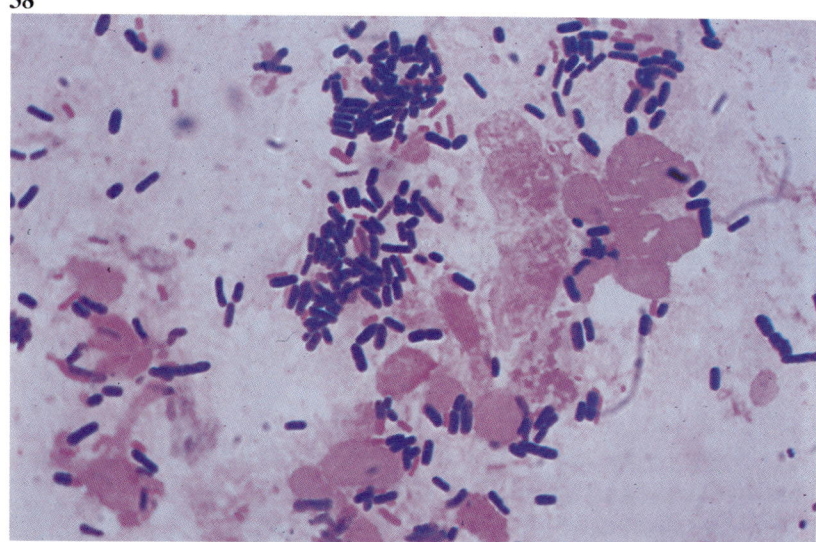

39 Necrosis of the inner part (arrows) of the small intestinal mucosa.

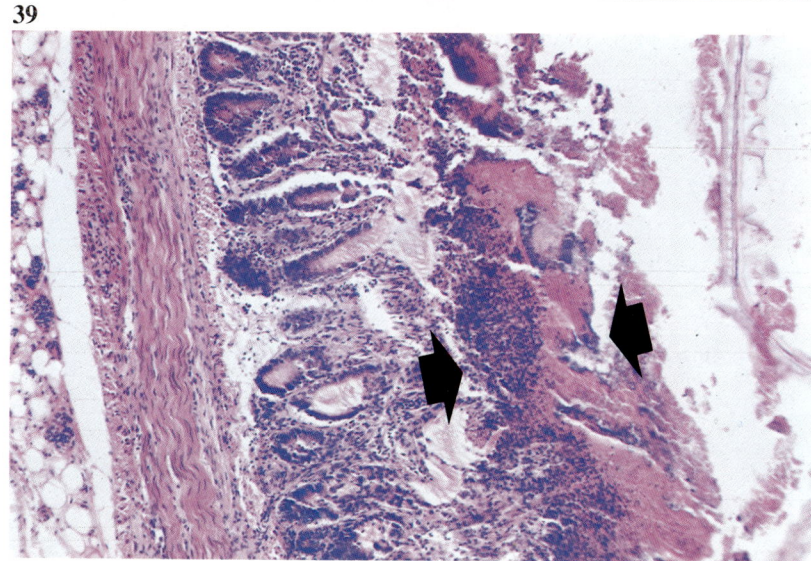

40 This section has been stained by the Gram-Weigart method. Numerous Gram-positive organisms are visible on the inner surface of the necrotic mucosa (right). The pink line (arrows) represents the junction of the inner necrotic tissue from the still viable deeper mucosa.

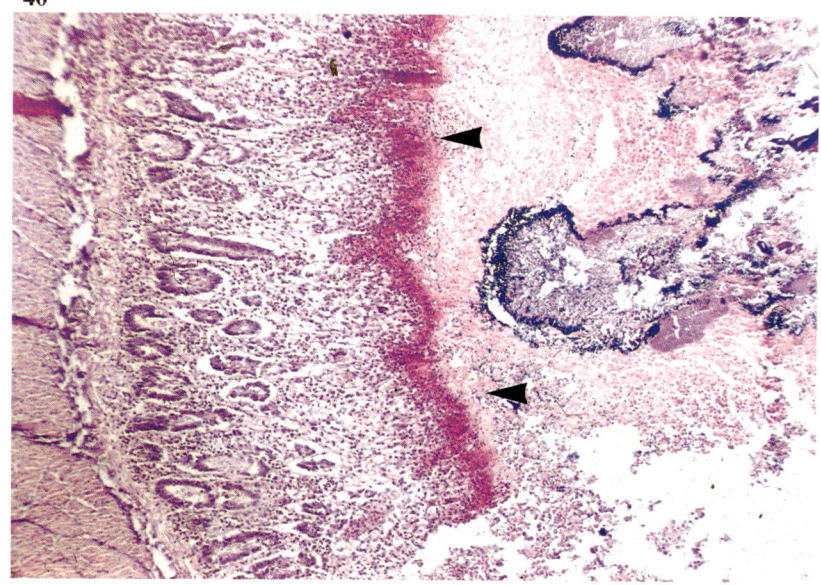

41 Kidneys of birds that have died as a result of necrotic enteritis are usually pale. This feature is often encountered in bacterial septicaemias and toxaemias and may give rise to the false impression that primary renal disease is present. Histologically, few changes are seen other than mild dilation of the distal parts of nephrons which is interpreted as a terminal dysfunction with, possibly, urates collecting in the distal tubules.

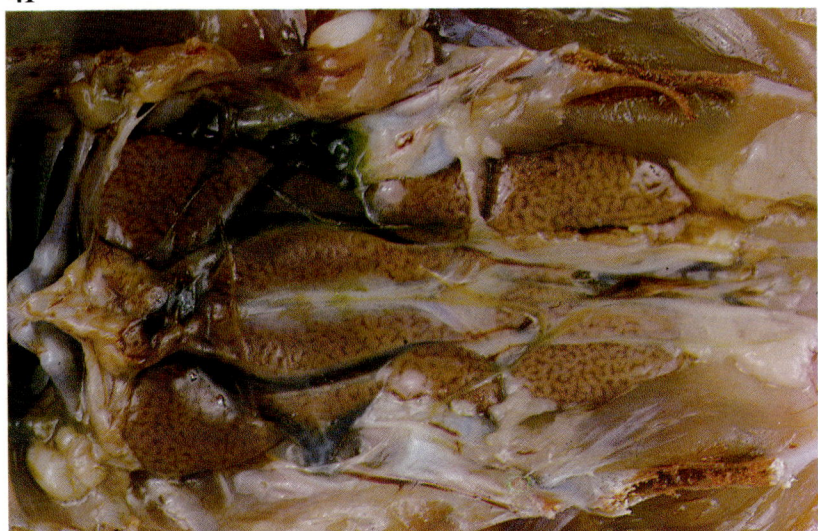

41

42 Intense congestion of a broiler liver. This degree of congestion is typical of acute cases. In some instances clostridia invade the portal blood system *post mortem* with the result that autolysis is more advanced in the tissue surrounding the intrahepatic veins, which causes mottling.

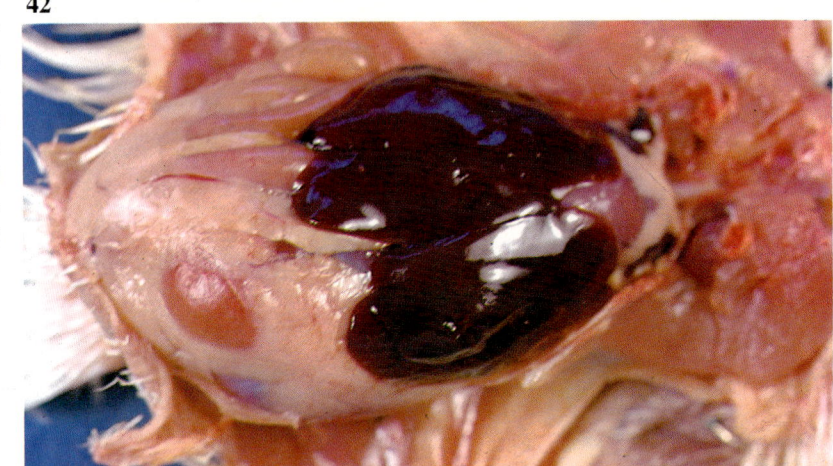

42

Gangrenous dermatitis

43 A small area of wet inflamed skin is present on this broiler's wing. Lesions like this are variable in size and may be present anywhere on the body. The condition is usually associated with either single or mixed infections of coagulase positive staphylococci and clostridia (eg *Cl. septicum* and *Cl. perfringens*). During the early part of an outbreak birds may die without obvious lesions affecting the skin but in some instances small wet sores can be found between the toes. Birds are rarely seen ill. If clostridia are involved the rate of decomposition of carcasses may be very rapid with the result that 'green' carcasses can be submitted with the history that the birds have been picked up as freshly dead an hour or two beforehand.

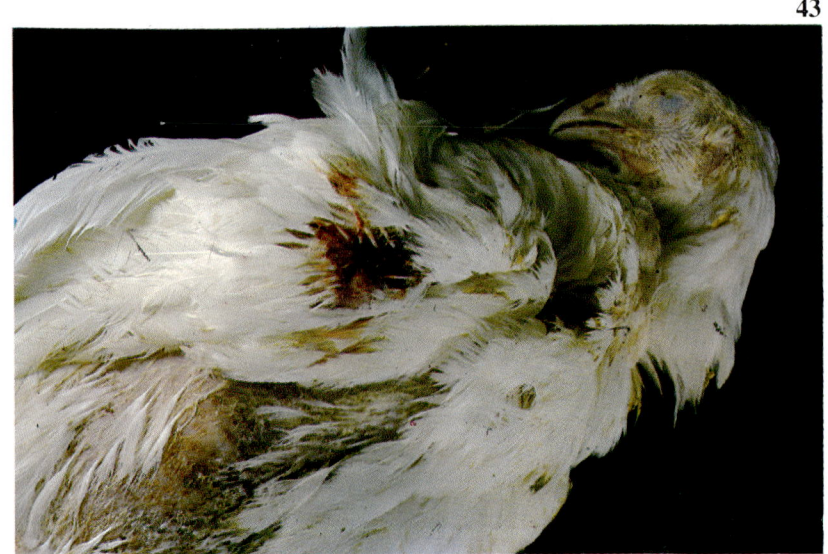

43

44 The skin lesions defeather very easily and are usually underrun with gelatinous and sanguinous fluid.

45 Part or all of the lung may undergo liquefaction. This is particularly common when the infection is predominantly staphylococcal. It may be the most notable post-mortem feature of carcasses examined at the beginning of outbreaks. Note the small unaffected areas of tissue at either end.

46 Clumps of staphylococci in a necrotic zone of lung.

44

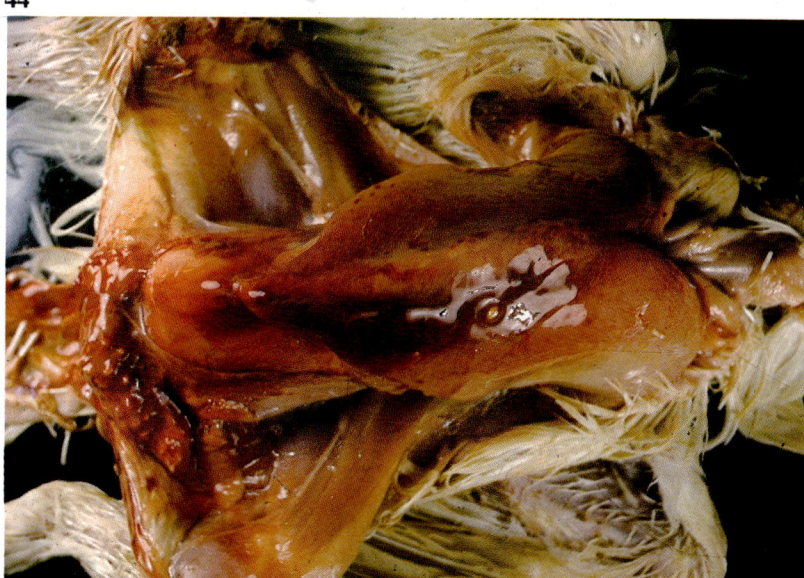

45

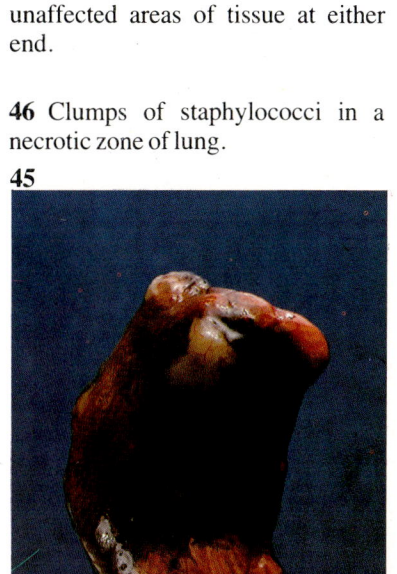

46

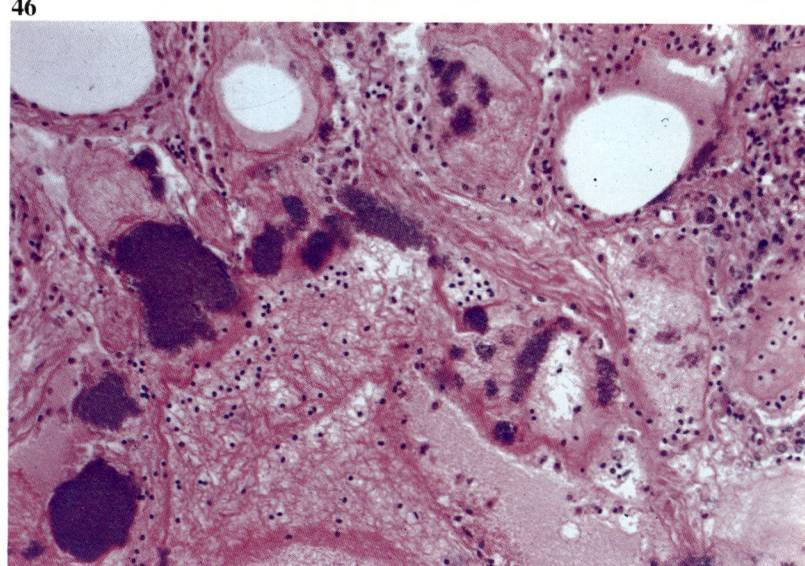

Listeriosis *(Listeria monocytogenes)*

47 Myocarditis in a 7-week-old commercial layer pullet. The heart has been cut through to show almost complete replacement of the myocardium with pale inflammatory tissue. Focal lesions may occur. The condition is uncommon and should not be confused with lymphoproliferative lesions of Marek's disease that often affect the heart, this is particularly so when necrosis has occurred in the lymphoid tumour giving rise to yellowish foci within the neoplasm.

47

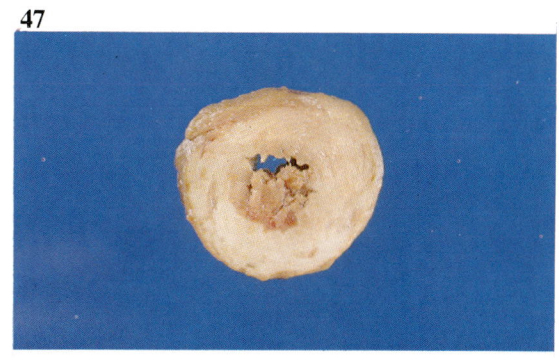

Erysipelas

(Erysipelothrix rhusiopathiae)

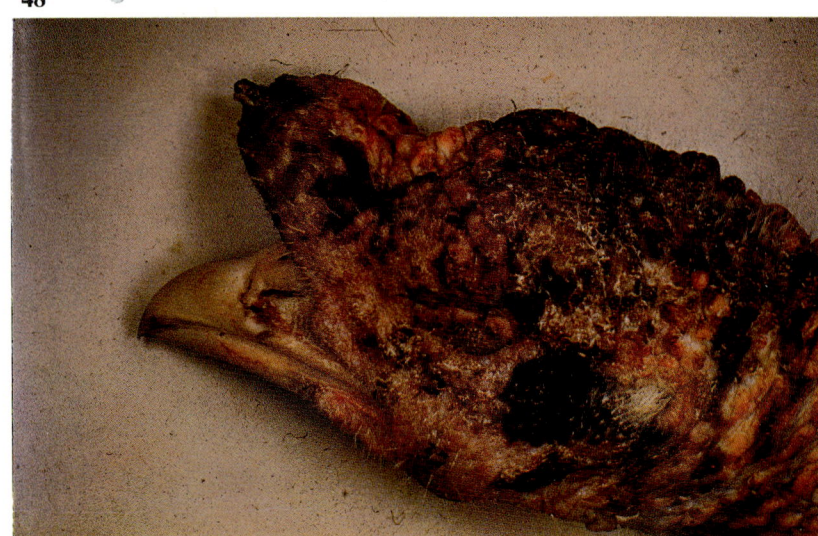

48 The condition is common in turkeys but rare in the fowl. Carcasses are congested and show general septicaemic changes. The head of this bird is scabbed. Gram-stained smears of the liver, kidney and bone marrow can be useful diagnostically if treatment has to be started immediately. In smears from tissue, the short rods tend to be more robust and strongly Gram-positive when compared to those made from cultures.

49 The livers of affected turkeys may have a distinctive par-boiled appearance.

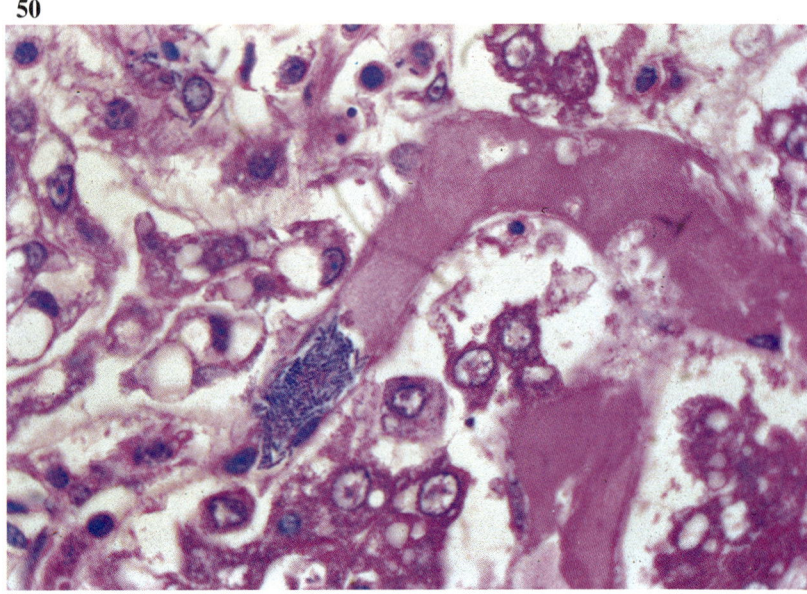

50 A clump of *E. rhusiopathiae* in a sinusoid of the liver shown in **49**. The sinusoidal disruption is partly artifactual. Acrylic resin.

Tuberculosis *(Mycobacterium avium)*

51 The disease is common in free range fowl but is only rarely seen under intensive systems of husbandry. Affected birds gradually become emaciated. Yellowish caseous nodules are most commonly found in the liver, spleen and intestine. Well developed lesions in the liver can usually be shelled out from the surrounding parenchyma.

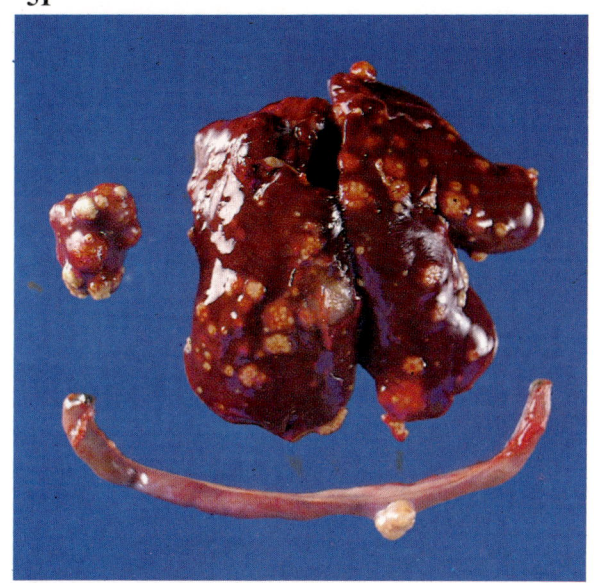

52 A pale granuloma within the marrow cavity of a femur. Lameness often occurs in affected birds due to the development of such lesions, particularly at the distal end of the femur.

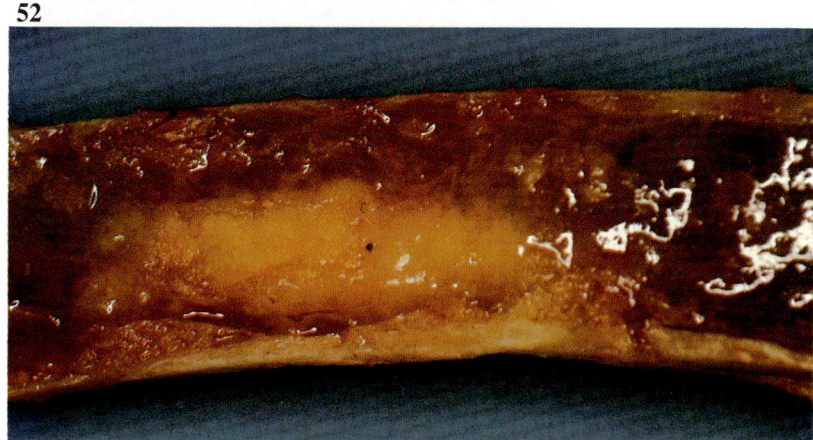

53 Large numbers of acid fast bacilli are present in smears from most avian lesions. Smears are best made by crushing individual nodules between two glass slides. Ziehl-Neelson.

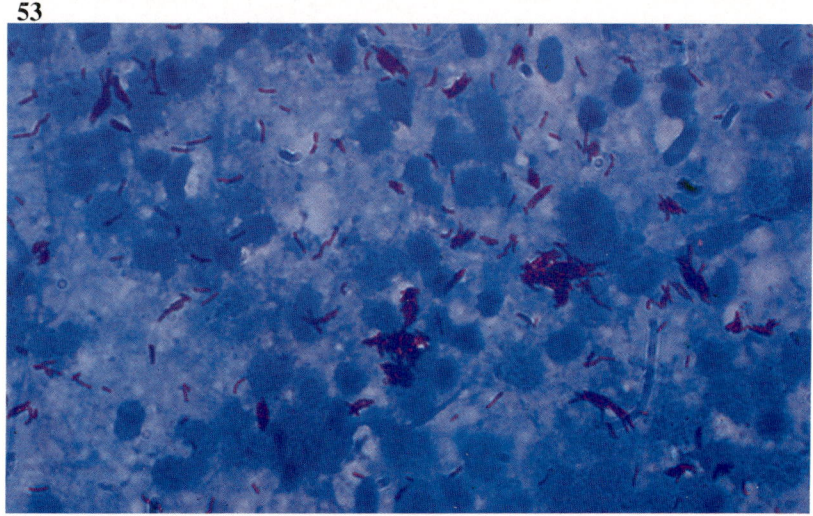

54 Developing tubercle in liver of hen. At this stage the central part of the lesion is mainly composed of pale-staining epithelioid cells.

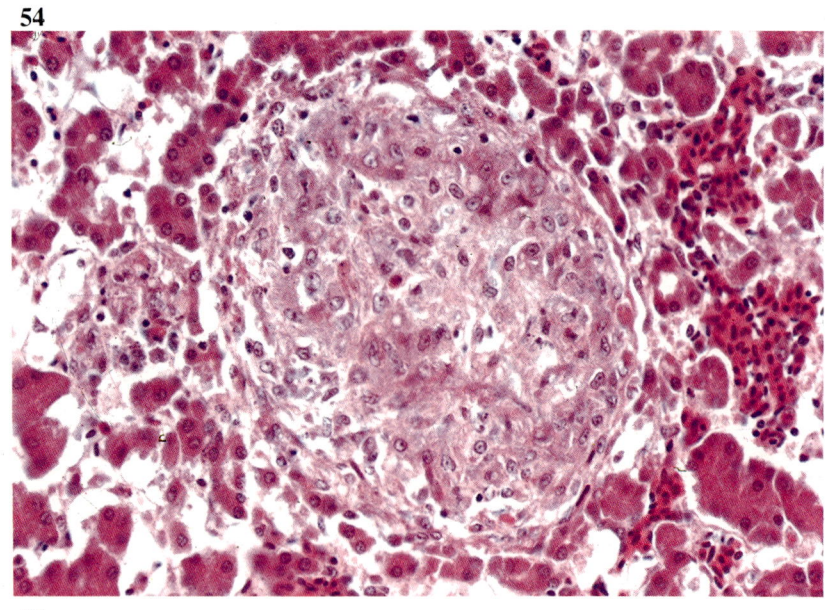

55 A more advanced lesion in which central necrosis has taken place. Giant cells are starting to pallisade round the necrotic zone. Numerous macrophages are present peripherally. Connective tissue encapsulation has not yet occurred.

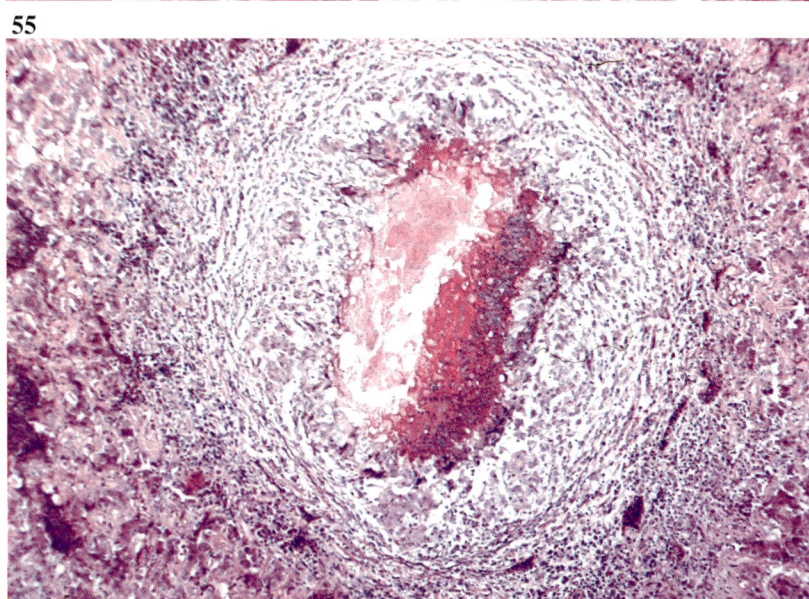

56 A large mass of granulation tissue was present at the thoracic inlet of a commercial layer. Many giant cells were scattered through the lesion in which there was considerable deposition of amyloid. A giant cell is seen engulfing an amyloid focus.

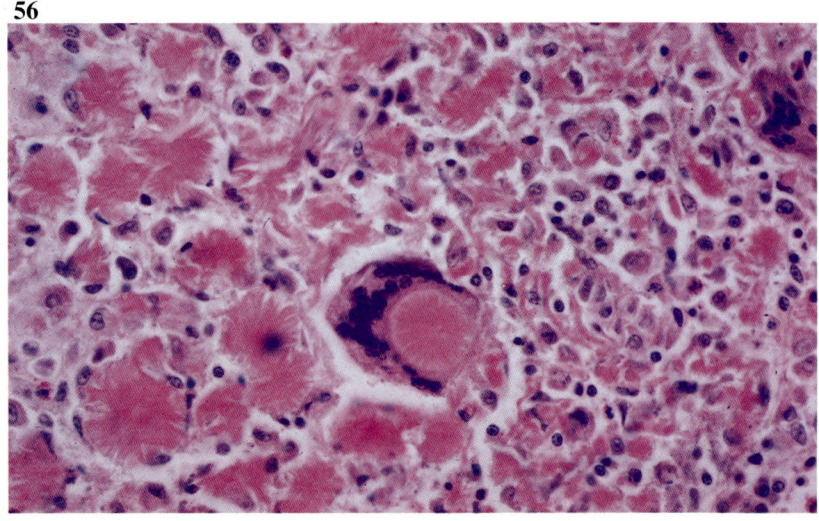

57 A Congo Red stain on the tissue in **56** demonstrates the characteristic apple-green birefringence of amyloid under polarised light.

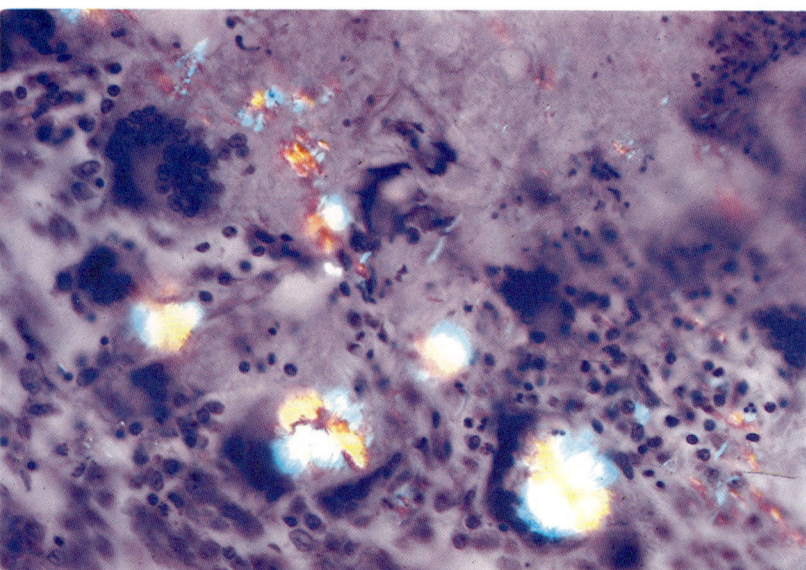

Vibrionic hepatitis

58 This condition is now rare and when seen is usually in young pullets. The livers may be enlarged and friable. Numerous small pale lesions are seen here under the capsule of a discoloured liver.

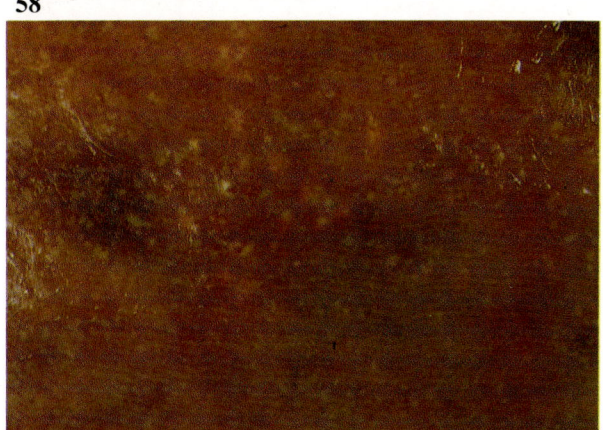

Salmonellosis

This section refers only to diseased birds. Many birds may be infected with salmonellas and show no clinical or post-mortem signs. As used here, the term 'salmonellosis' also refers to the now rare diseases caused by *Salmonella pullorum* and *S. gallinarum*.

59 *Salmonella typhimurium*. Gross lesions are very variable. Heavy mortality may result in young chicks and turkey poults. Focal lesions are present in the liver of this 7-day-old broiler. In birds of a few weeks of age the gross lesions may occasionally resemble those of Coli septicaemia (*see* **1**). Histologically, diagnoses of meningitis are made from time to time in young chicks with clinical histories of nervous signs.

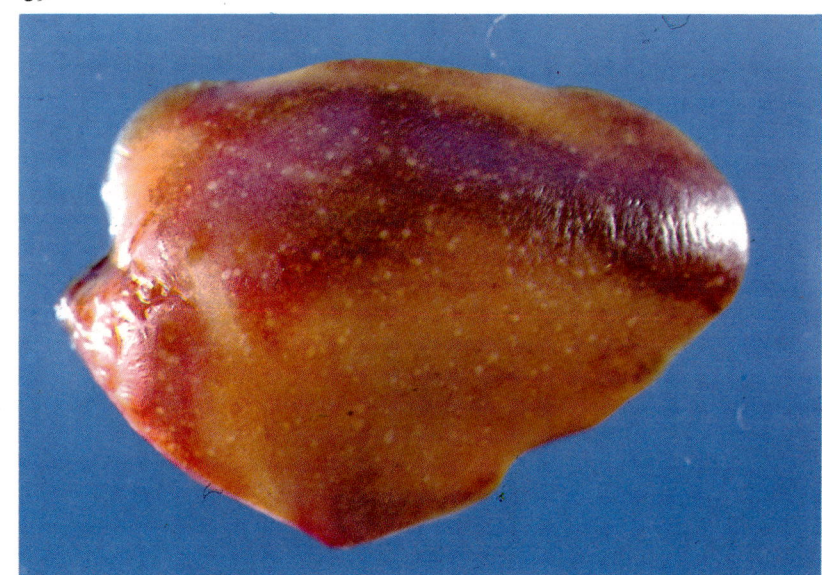

60

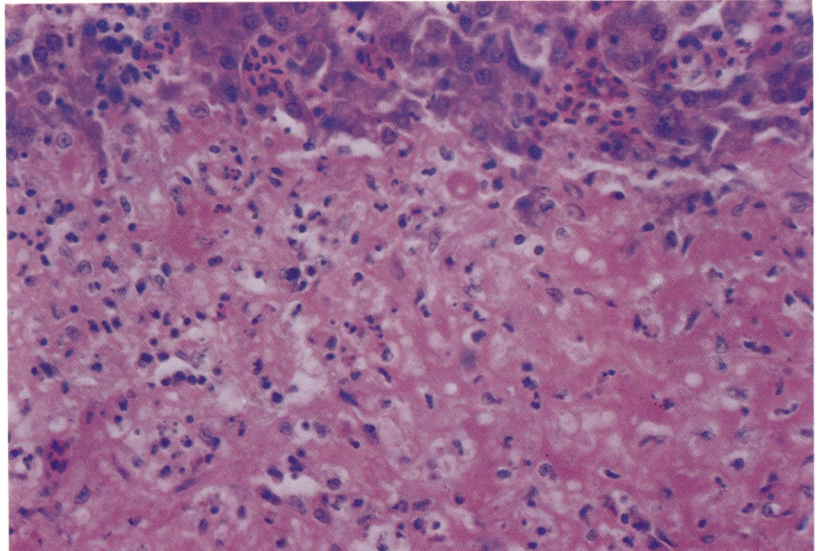

61

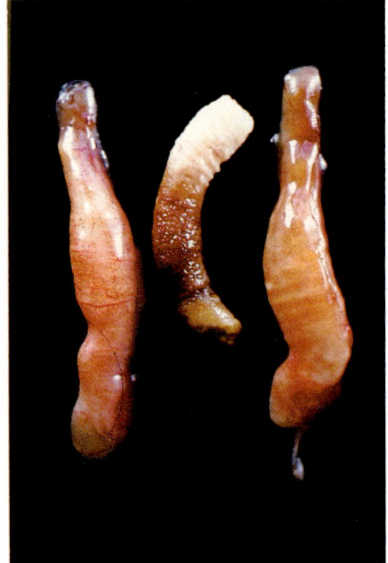

62

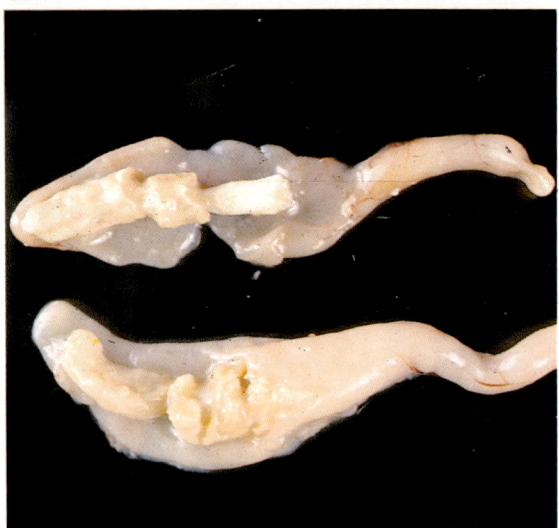

63

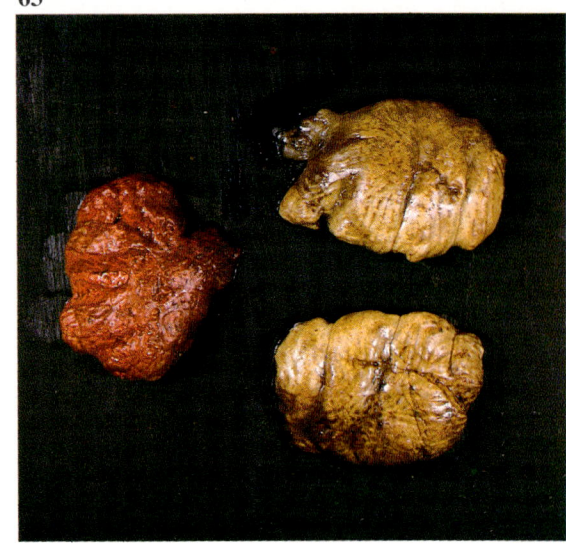

60 *S. typhimurium*. A section of liver from **59**. Necrotic tissue in one of the focal lesions is in the lower part of the photograph and is staining more eosinophilically than the unaffected hepatocytes above.

61 *S. typhimurium*. Vermiform appearance of the caeca resulting from an acute typhlitis in a 7-day-old broiler. The presence of this lesion is variable but salmonella infection should be suspected when it is seen.

62 *S. typhimurium*. Cheesy cores of inflammatory debris within the caeca of a boiler chick.

63 *S. gallinarum* (fowl typhoid). In most acute cases the lungs show a brown discolouration.

64 *S. gallinarum*. The carcases of birds that have died from the acute disease are jaundiced and the liver shows a characteristic bronzing (right) after exposure to the air. Note also the severe congestion of the spleen.

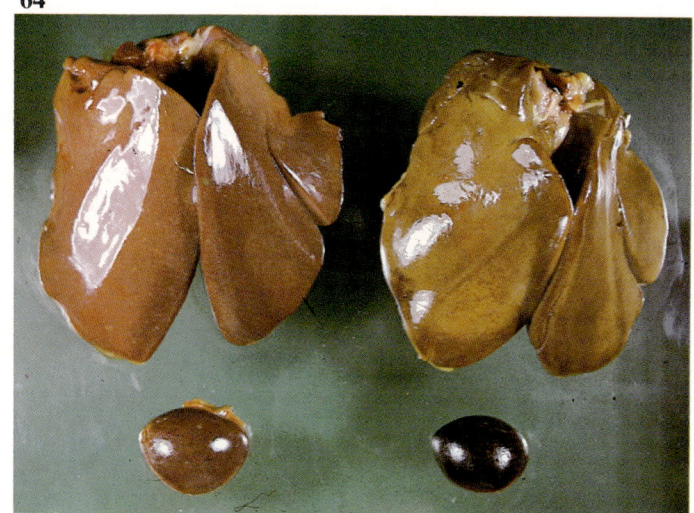

65 *S. pullorum* (bacillary white diarrhoea). Greyish-white necrotic foci in chick lung. Similar lesions may be present in the heart and liver.

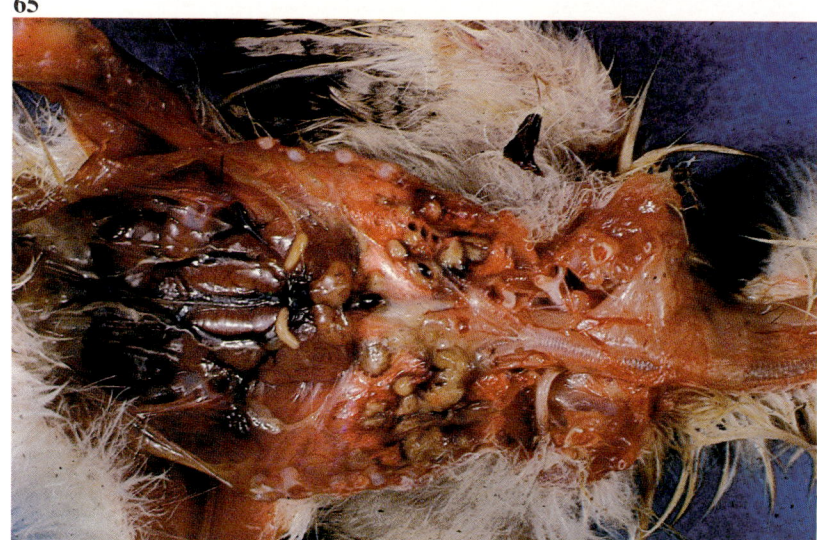

66 *S. pullorum*. Synovitis of hock joints in chicks.

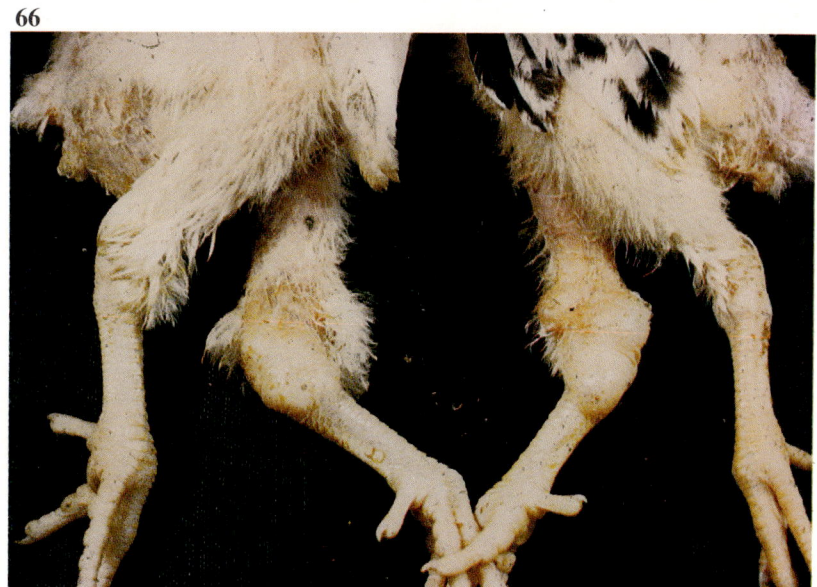

67 *S. pullorum.* In adults, the ovary is the organ most frequently involved. This specimen shows a few degenerate ova, some of which are attached to the body of the organ by long stalks. The contents of the affected ova are discoloured and may be inspissated.

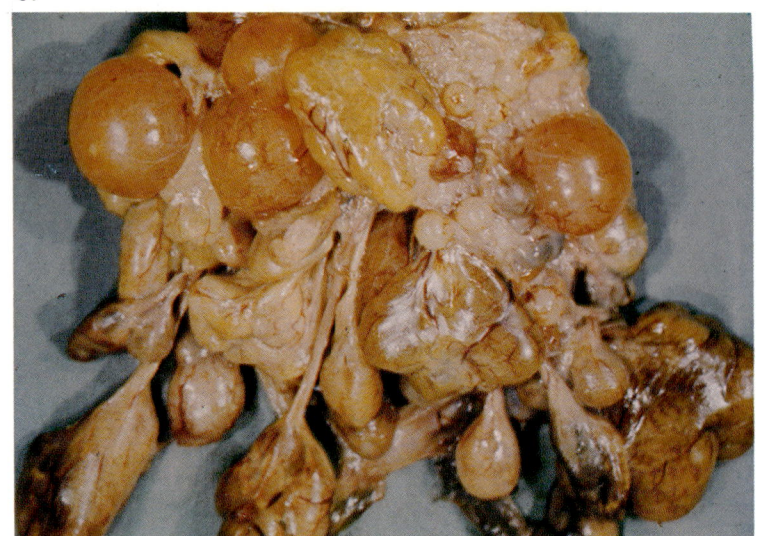

Mycoplasmosis

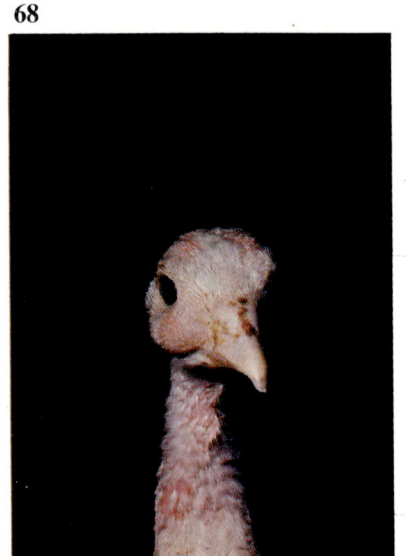

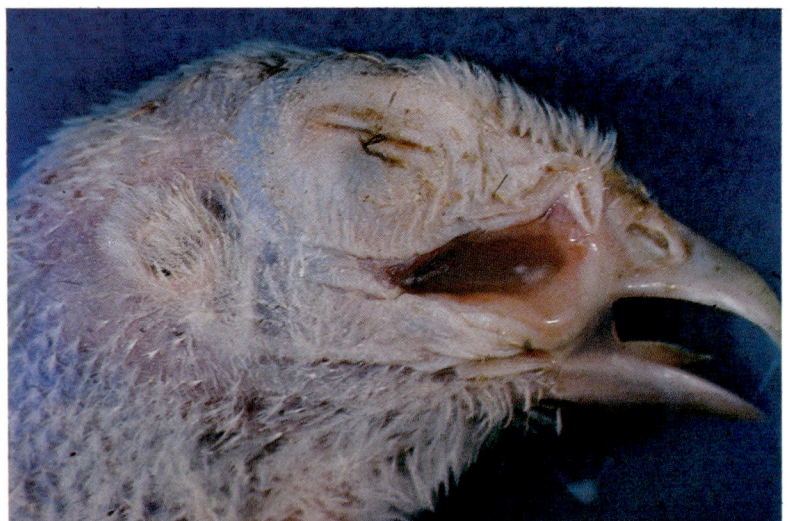

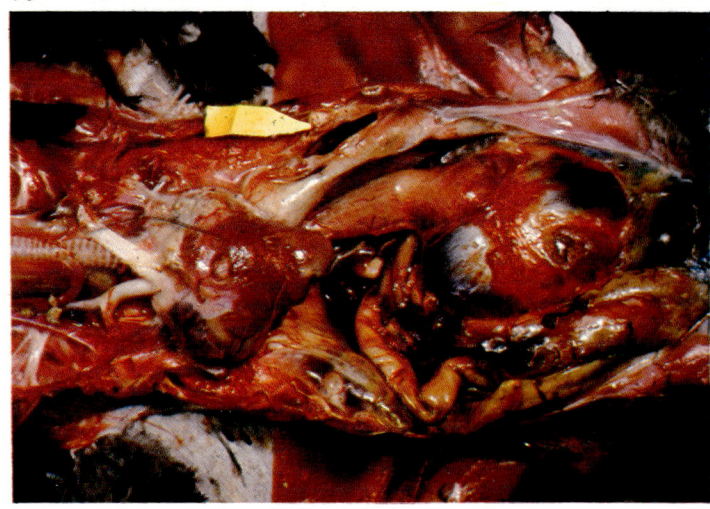

68 *M. gallisepticum.* Swelling of the infra-orbital sinuses in a turkey.

69 *M. gallisepticum.* Infra-orbital sinus of a turkey opened to show sticky exudate in an acute case.

70 *M. gallisepticum.* Gross lesions tend to be more pronounced in the turkey and infection is often accompanied by air sacculitis (yellow pointer) and pneumonia.

71 *M. gallisepticum.* Pneumonia associated with infection in a turkey. The inflammatory exudate is mixed.

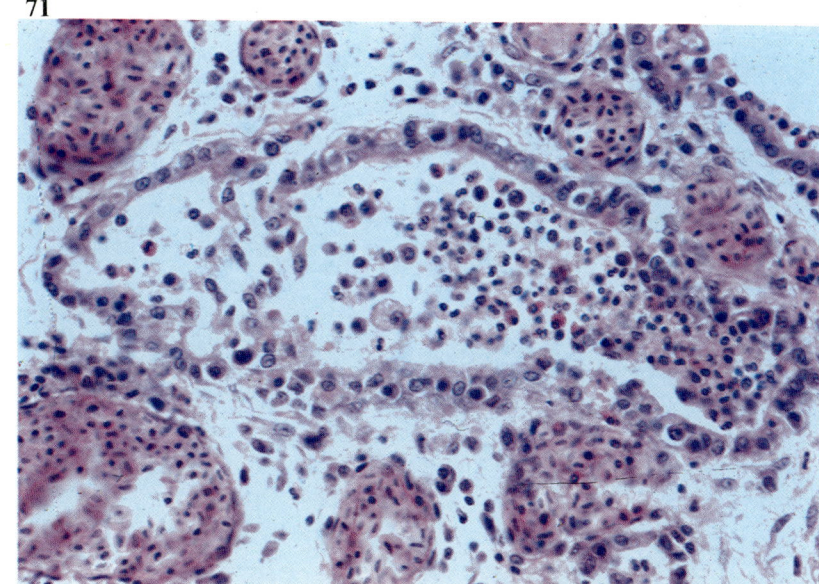

72 *M. synoviae* (infectious synovitis). Subcutaneous bursitis over the sternum in a 9-week-old commercial layer pullet. Note the loss of condition. (*NB M. synoviae* may be associated with respiratory disease complexes in broilers; joint and bursal lesions in such flocks are usually absent.)

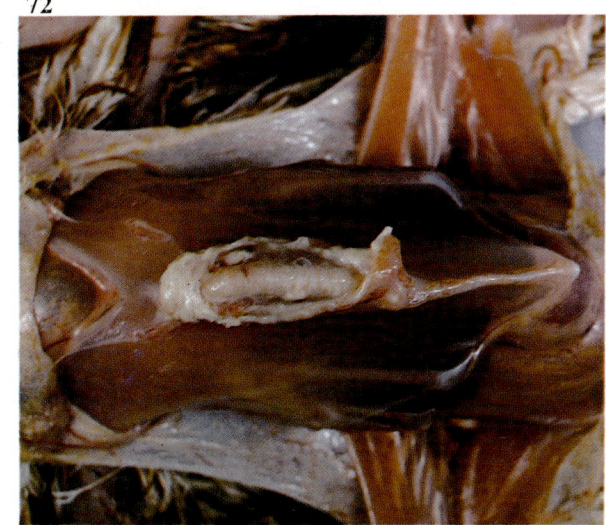

73 *M. synoviae.* Two swollen footpads (centre and left) of broilers. This feature may be very pronounced. There is frequently swelling of the hock and main wing joints. As in other mycoplasma infections, egg transmission occurs and the diagnosis should be carefully confirmed, both serologically and culturally.

74 *M. synoviae.* Footpad exudate in an acute infection of a commercial layer. The exudate is characteristically glairy and tenacious.

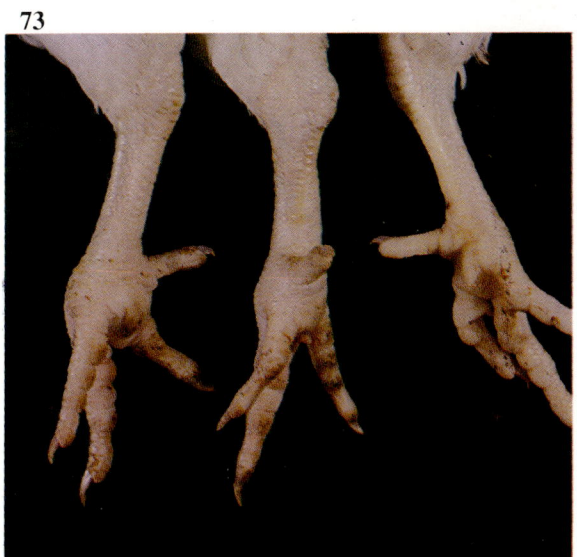

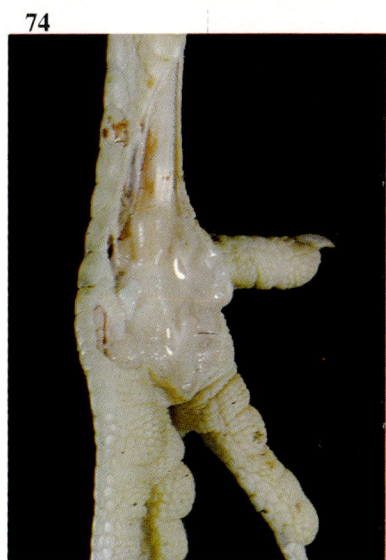

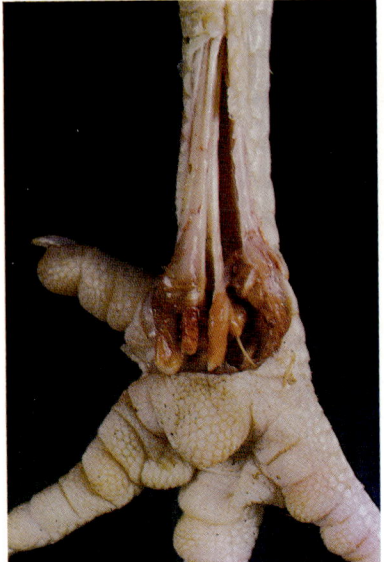

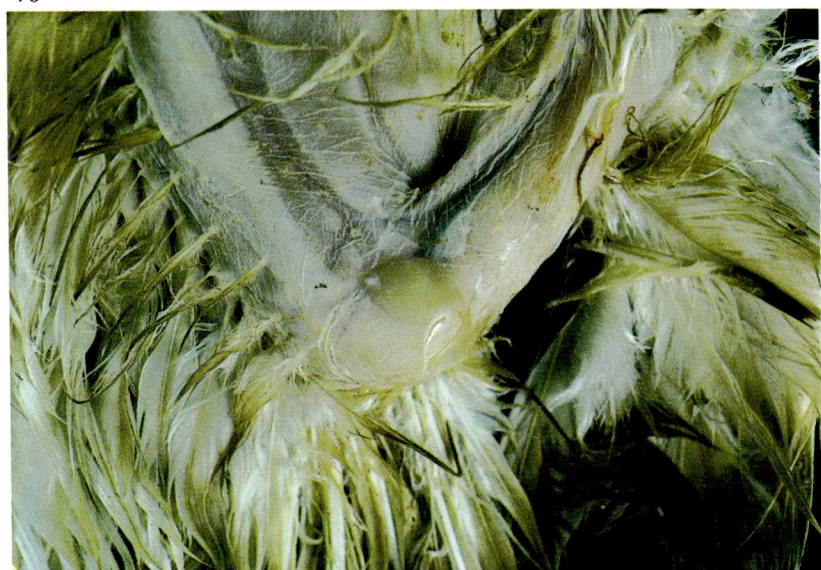

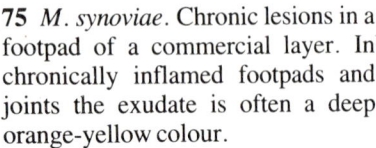

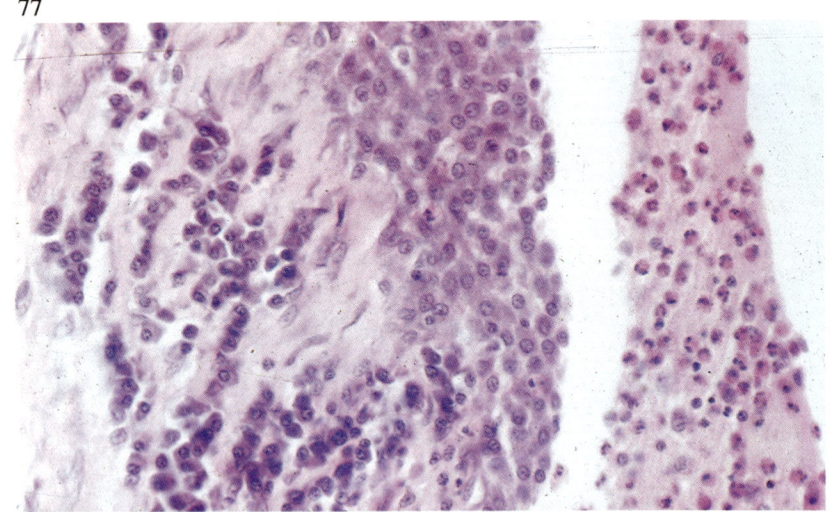

75 *M. synoviae*. Chronic lesions in a footpad of a commercial layer. In chronically inflamed footpads and joints the exudate is often a deep orange-yellow colour.

76 *M. synoviae*. An inflamed wing joint has been opened to demonstrate the exudate. Inflammation of wing joints is occasionally seen in staphylococcal infections but infectious synovitis should always be suspected when lesions are being encountered frequently in this joint and accompanied by sternal bursitis.

77 *M. synoviae*. Purulent exudate to the right of a chronically inflamed synovial membrane.

78 *M. meleagridis*. Infection may cause poor growth and feathering, chondrodystrophy, air sacculitis and diarrhoea (turkey syndrome '65). The legs of this turkey have a severe varus deformity at the hock joint.

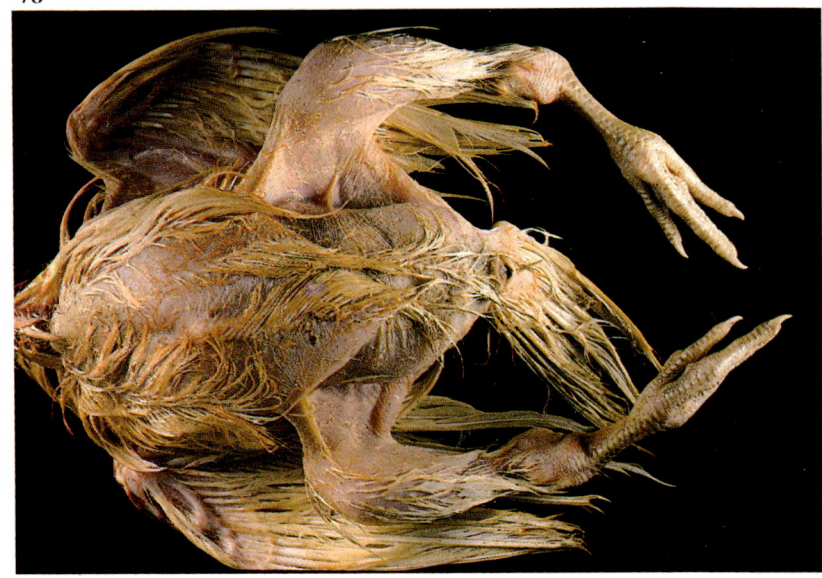

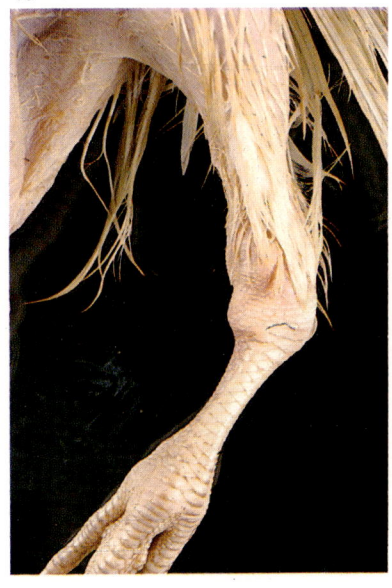

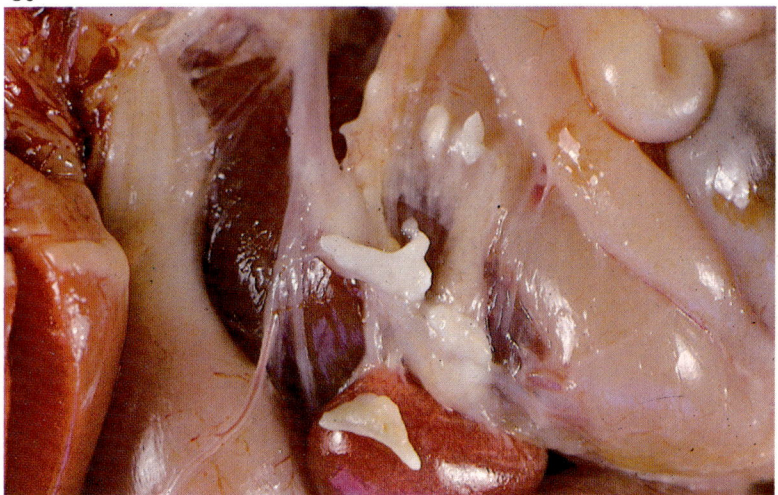

79 *M. meleagridis.* Closer view of a chondrodystrophic tarso-metatarsus in the same bird as shown in **78**. Note the shortening and flattening of the proximal head.

80 *M. meleagridis.* Flecks of caseous exudate within the abdominal air sacs of a 6-week-old turkey.

81 *M. meleagridis.* Section of a widened head of an affected tarsometatarsus. Martius scarlet blue.

82 *M. meleagridis.* Paucity of developing chondrocytes with some necrosis (arrows) in the transitional zone of the growth plate seen in **81**. Martius scarlet blue.

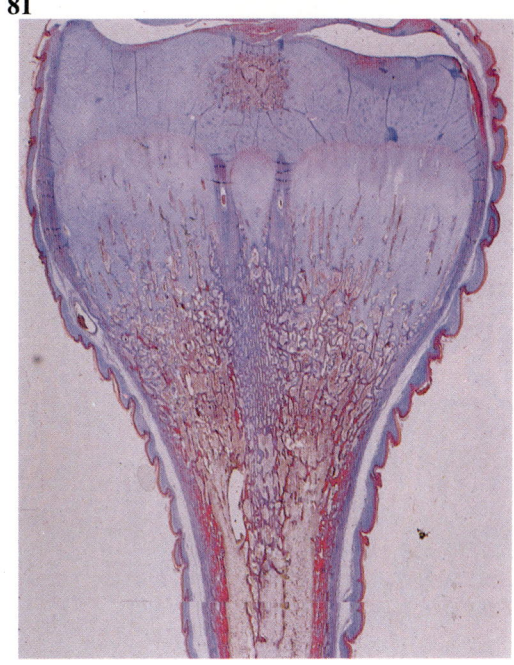

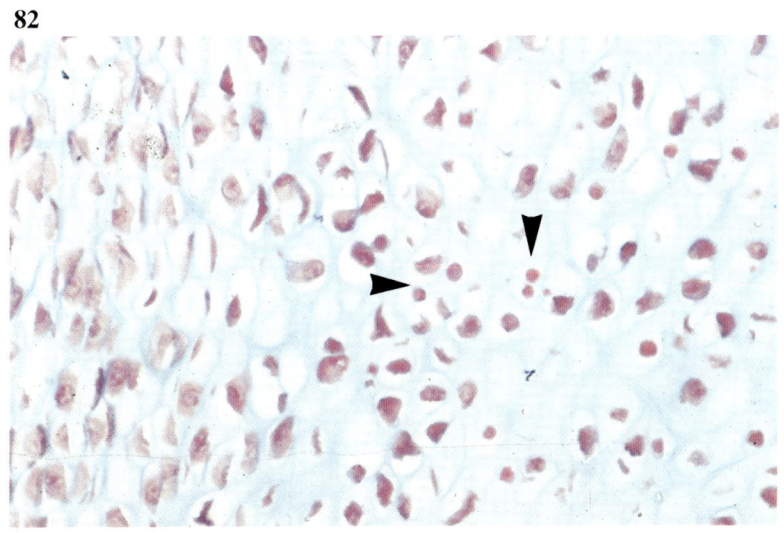

Viral diseases

Infectious bursal disease (Gumboro disease)

83 The bursa of Fabricius is slightly swollen in this 3-week-old broiler. The small highlight on the surface has been produced by a thin layer of gelatinous oedema covering the serous surface. This infection was subclinical.

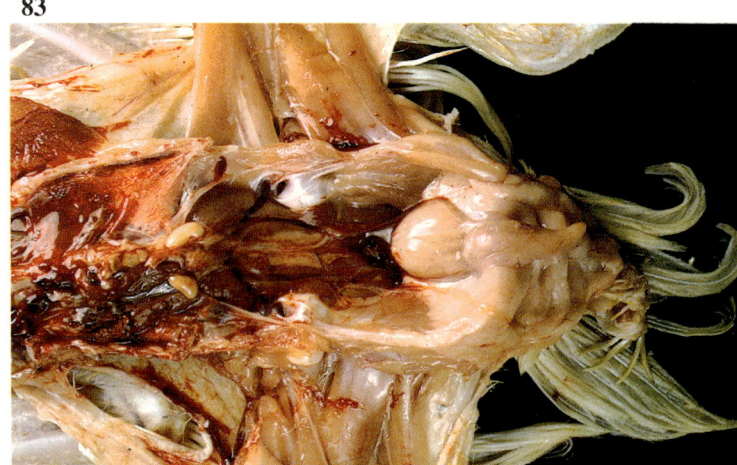

84 Swollen bursa of Fabricius in a clinical case.

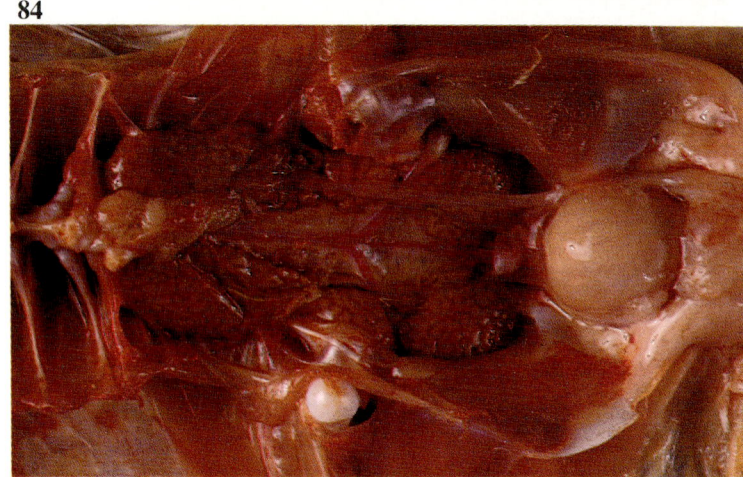

85 Haemorrhagic lesions are usually encountered in the bursa if mortality is occurring. Lesions vary in severity from a few petechial haemorrhages on the plicae to very severe haemorrhage, as here, throughout the organ. Purulent luminal exudate may become inspissated. The kidneys of birds that have died are often swollen and pale. This is caused by a terminal dysfunction and is not a nephritis.

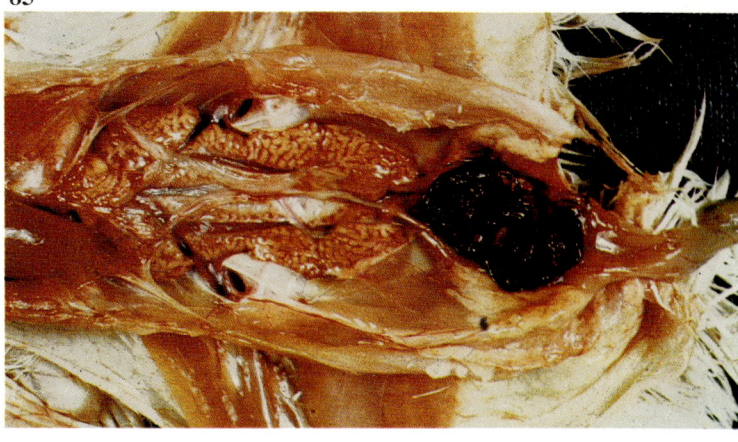

86 Extensive haemorrhages are present in the follicles and interfollicular tissue. Purulent exudate (arrow) has collected in the bursal lumen.

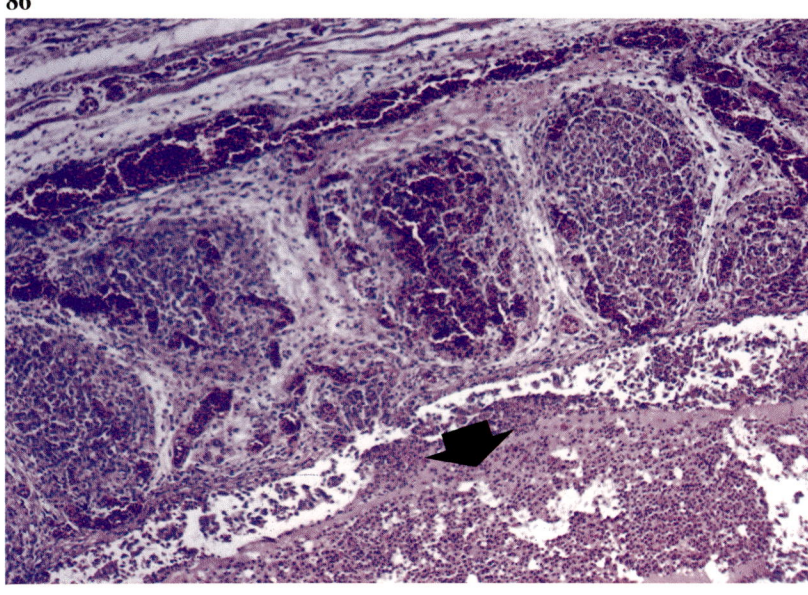

87 Sub-clinical disease. Bursal haemorrhages are not usually present but a higher power view of an injured follicle shows lymphocytolysis and heterophilic infiltration. Infectious bursal disease must be distinguished histologically from causes of *non-inflammatory* lymphoid depletion and premature bursal regression. This is readily done providing the lesions are observed during the early stages of the disease when the acute inflammatory reaction is evident.

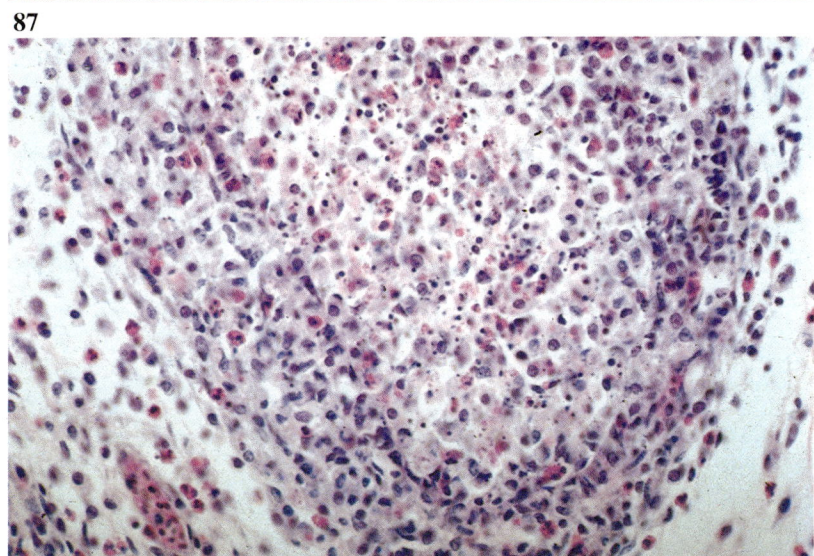

88 Cystic spaces forming in injured follicles. This may be a prominent feature during resolution. The acute inflammatory reaction is quickly cleared in most cases leaving severely depleted follicles and fibroplasia of the interfollicular connective tissue. Hyperplasia of the bursal epithelium is often marked at this stage.

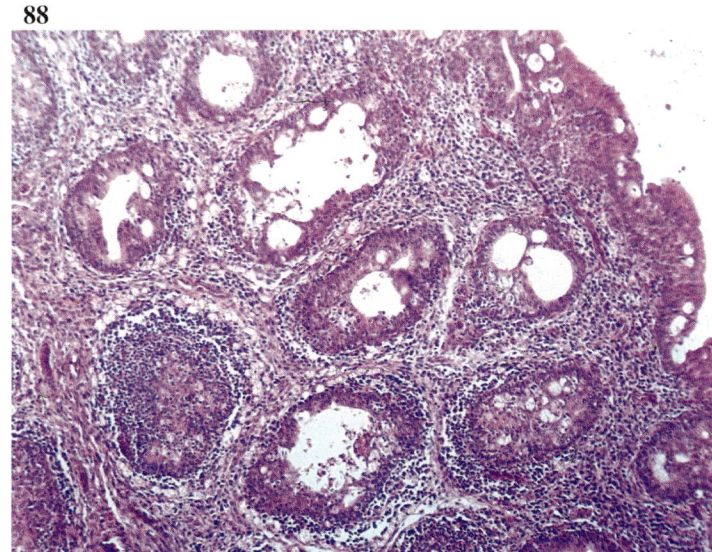

89 Small linear muscular haemorrhages may be present in birds that
have died. Although the pectoral
muscles are shown here, the outer
surface of the thigh is the site where
these lesions are most likely to occur.

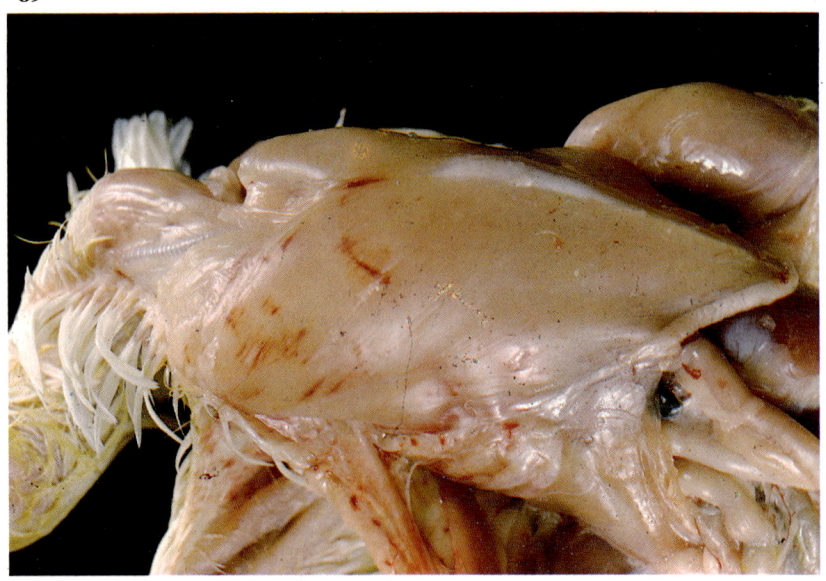

Inclusion body hepatitis

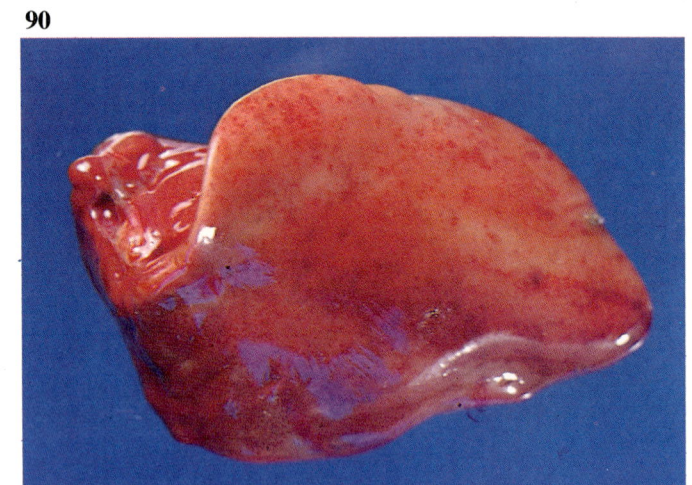

90 The disease is seen mainly in young broilers
and broiler breeders. The carcases are usually
congested and the livers may show characteristic
small speckled haemorrhages throughout the sub-
stance of the organ. In some cases, however, the
liver may be just swollen and pale. Gross lesions
may need to be distinguished from those of the
fatty liver kidney syndrome (*see* **216-224**).

91 The appearance of intranuclear
inclusions within hepatocytes is variable. In some cases these may be
almost entirely eosinophilic and well
haloed or they may be predominantly
basophilic and solid. If the lesions are
focal, inclusions tend to be seen near
their periphery.

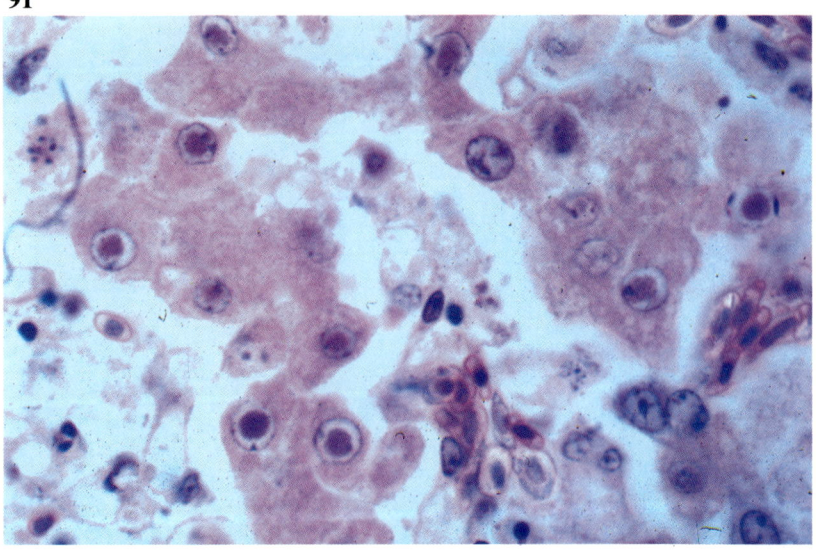

92 The kidneys are often congested and tinged a muddy yellow colour, possibly due to slight carcase jaundice.

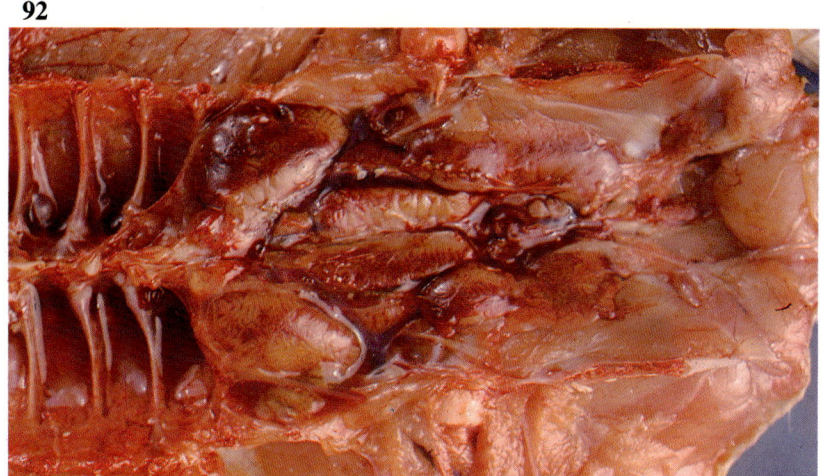

Haemorrhagic enteritis in turkeys

93 The small intestine is usually distended with blood and mucosal debris. The mucosa, particularly in the upper region, tends to have a velvety appearance. The spleens may be swollen and mottled.

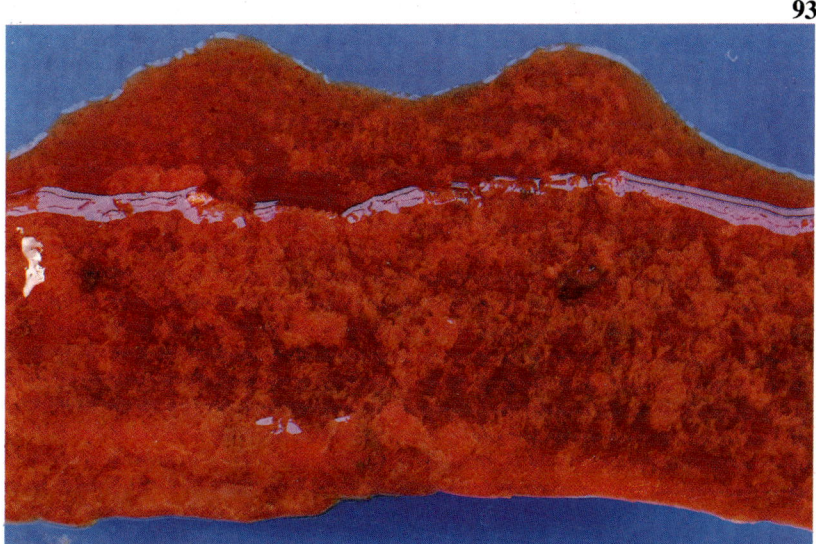

94 The presence of intranuclear inclusions (solid, pale-staining bodies are arrowed) within the intestinal lamina propria is a useful diagnostic feature. Acrylic resin.

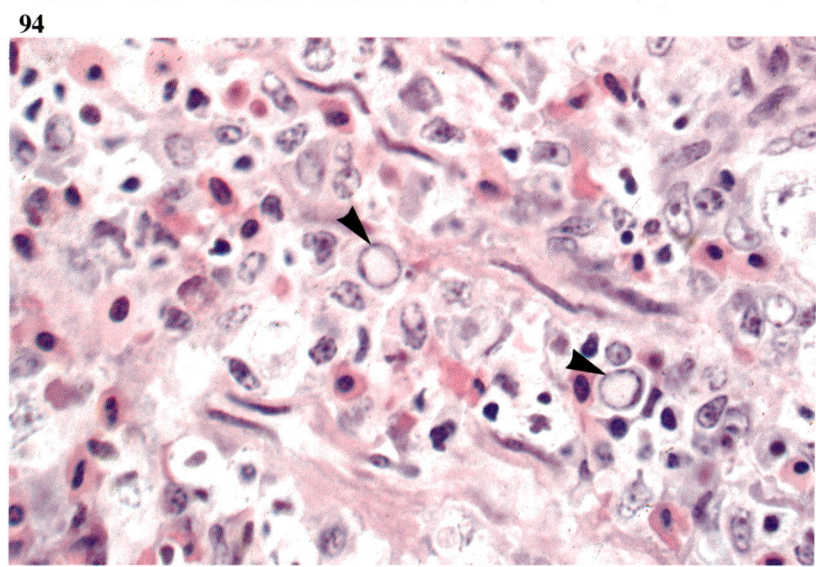

95 Numerous, similarly staining intranuclear inclusions (arrows) within the reticulum cells are visible in the spleen. Acrylic resin.

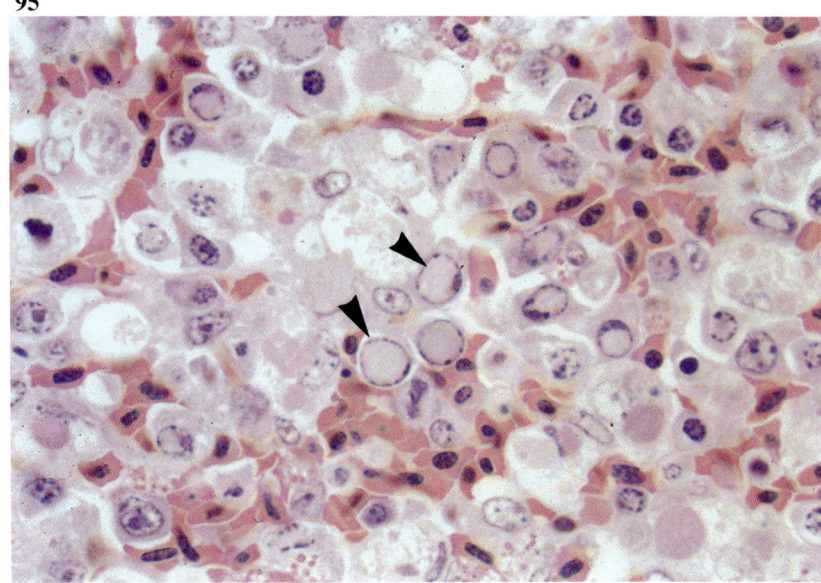

Fowl pox

96 The disease may affect both chickens and turkeys and can cause cutaneous and internal lesions. Here, pox lesions are present in the oropharynx of a hen. Lesions may also occur in the trachea and should be distinguished culturally and histophathologically from diphtheritic forms of ILT (*see* **99**). The disease is now seen infrequently but has appeared in some battery systems, both on its own and in combination with other infectious agents.

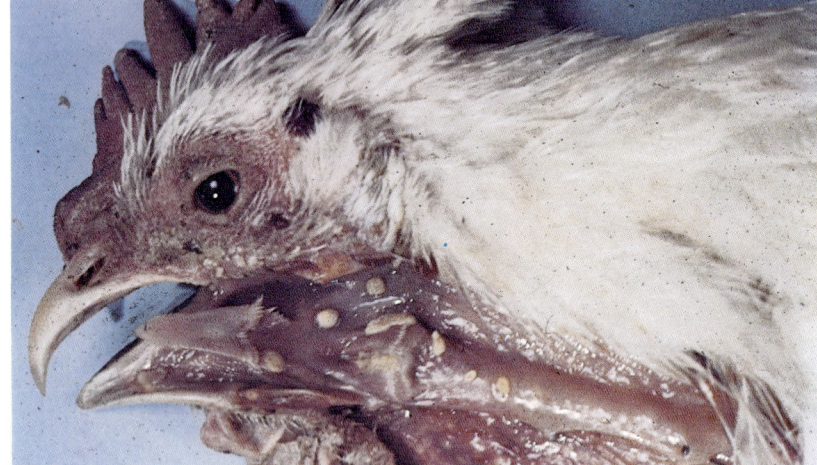

97 Large eosinophilic cytoplasmic inclusions in a proliferative epithelial lesion. Pigeon skin is shown here in order to demonstrate the typical avian pox lesion.

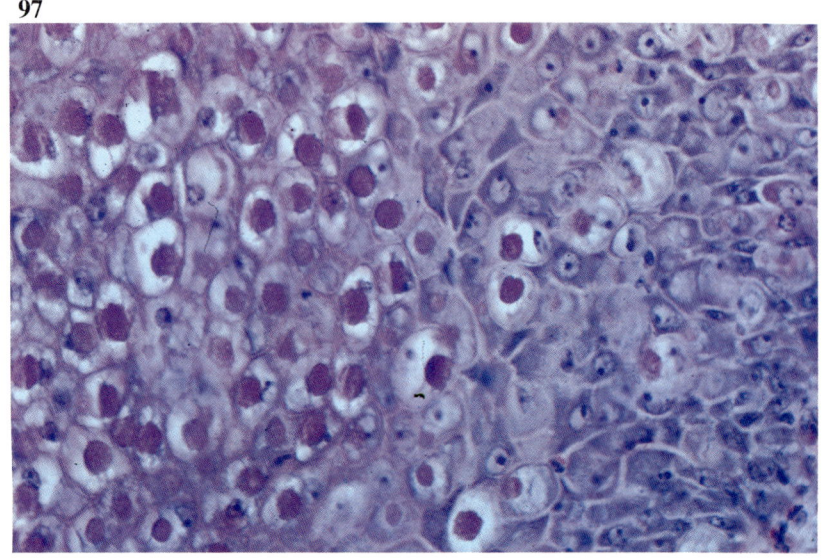

Infectious laryngotracheitis (ILT)

98 Lesions are confined to the respiratory tract. Post-mortem examination may show occlusion of the tracheal lumen with blood and blood clots.

98

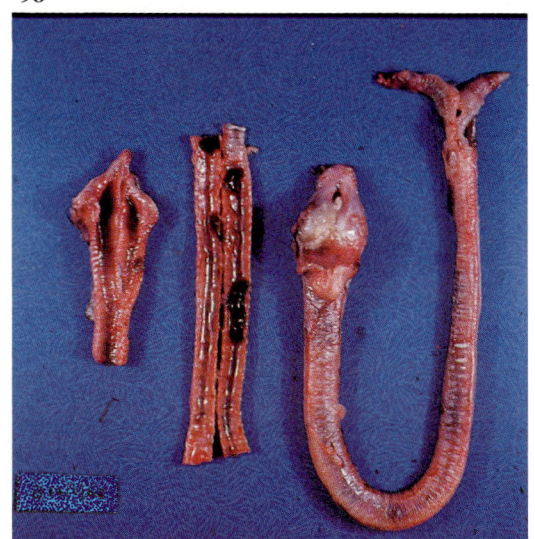

99 In more chronic forms of the disease there may be a pronounced diphtheresis in the trachea.

99

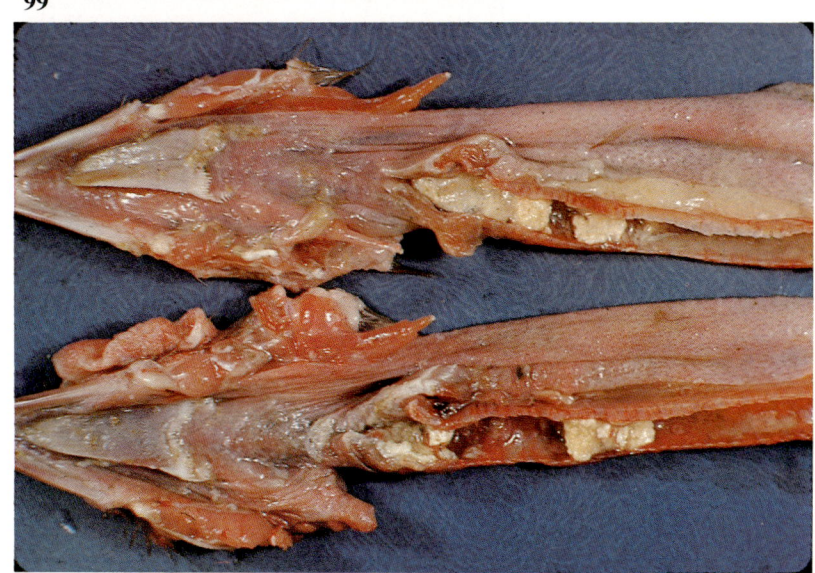

100 Two partly fixed broiler tracheas are compared. The one on the right is full of purulent debris, the other contains a blood clot.

100

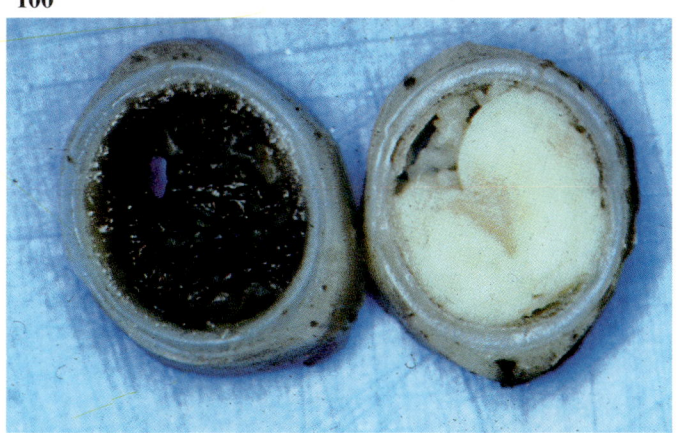

101 Eosinophilic intranuclear inclusions are present in a clump of epithelial cells that have been sloughed from the inflamed mucous membrane. These were lying in a large mass of inflammatory exudate within the lumen. Such clumps of cells may be quite small but often repay close examination. The inclusions may not necessarily be haloed and can therefore be more difficult to see. If groups of nuclei containing haloed inclusions are packed close together the margination of the chromatin can give a 'wire-netting' effect.

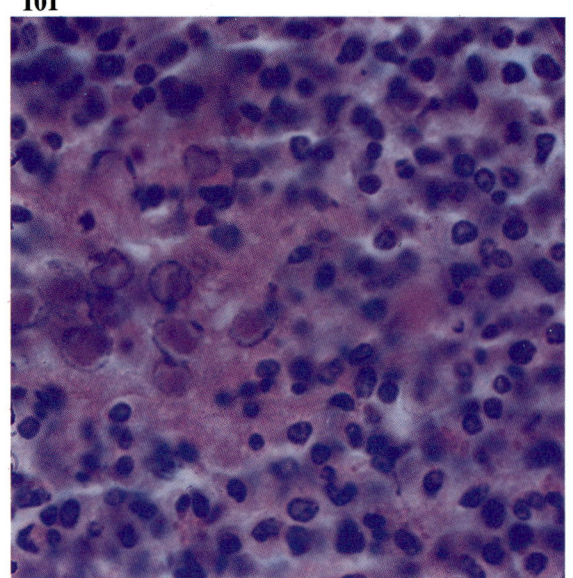

Newcastle disease

102 Depending on the strain of virus and its tissue tropism the post-mortem findings are very variable. Petechial haemorrhages are shown here on the heart and abdominal fat in a congested carcase of a fowl. Haemorrhages on the tracheal mucosa and air sacculitis may be seen with some pneumotropic strains of the virus.

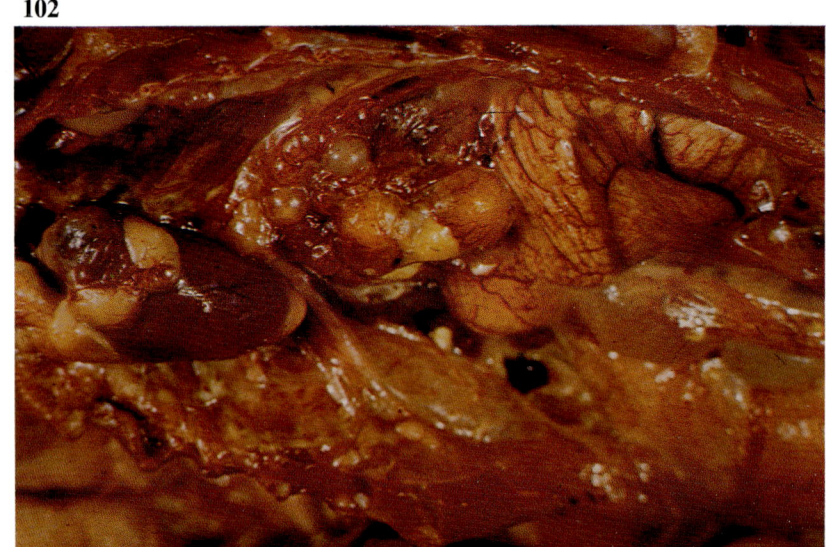

103 If present, proventricular haemorrhages are usually seen on the surface of the papillae and can be distributed in a ring near the junction with the gizzard. Haemorrhagic lesions may also be found in the intestine, particularly on the surface of the caecal 'tonsils'.

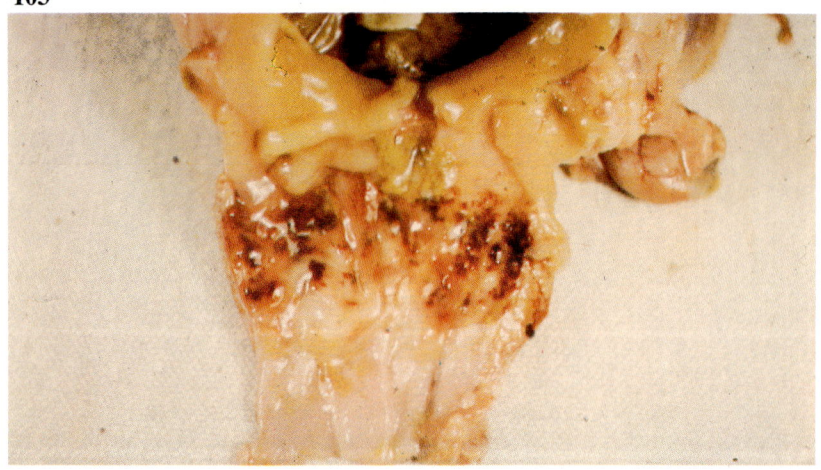

104 Submucosal oedema (arrow) in the trachea of an unvaccinated fowl. Inflammation has resulted in most of the epithelium being shed, leaving small protruding pegs of tunica propria. The lesion is not specific but was observed during outbreaks involving a pneumotropic strain of the virus.

104

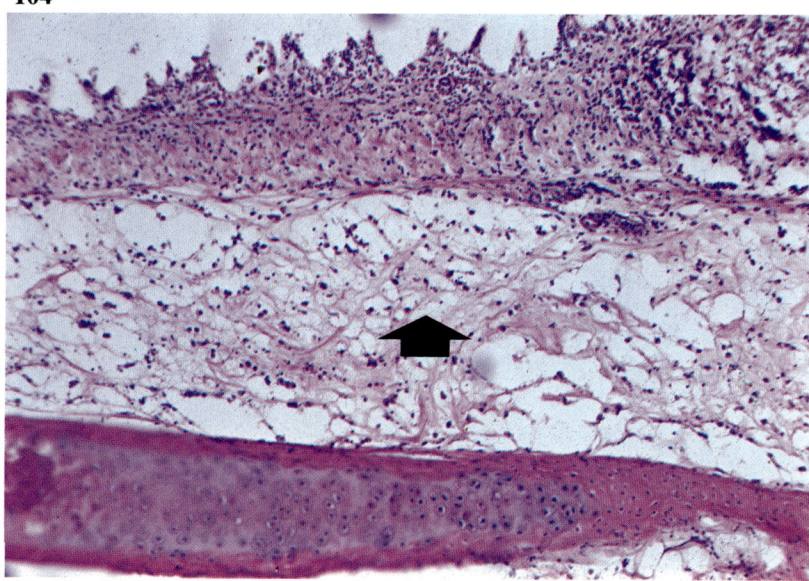

105 Non-purulent encephalitis may be present. In this photograph localised gliosis (arrows) involves the molecular layer of the cerebellum in a fowl.

105

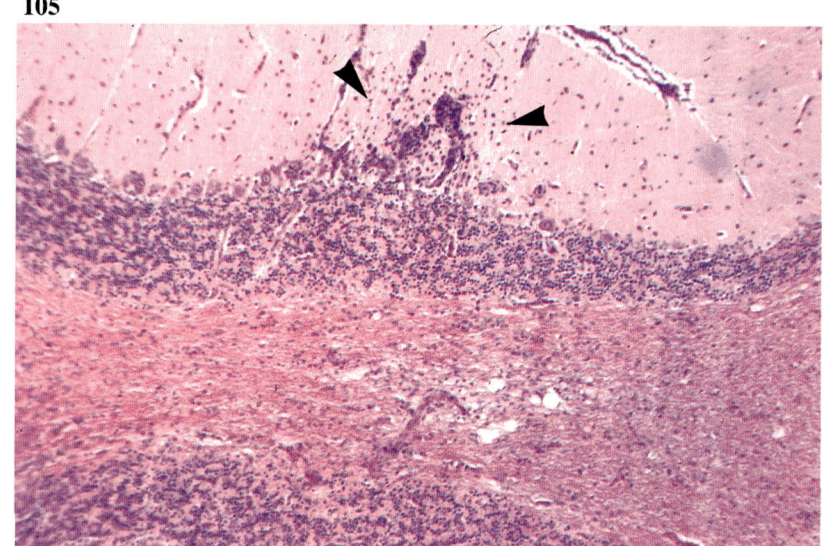

106 Perivascular cuffing in a section of cerebrum from a fowl.

106

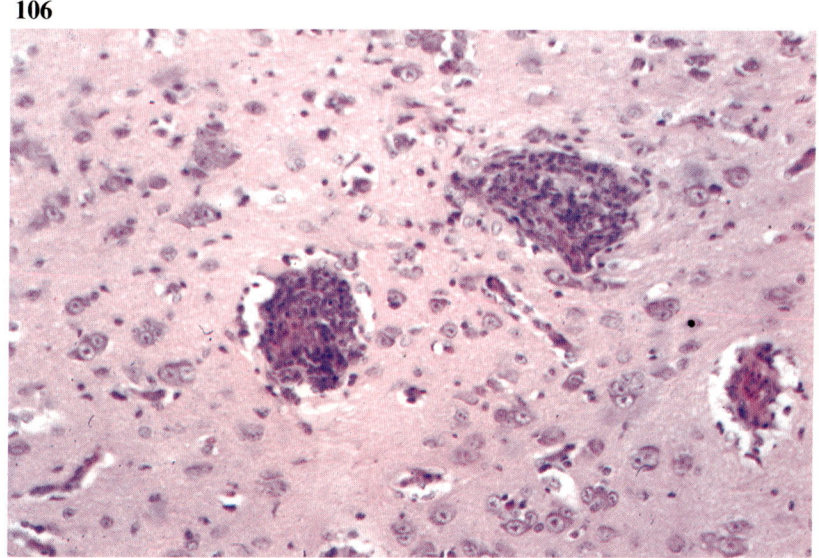

Infectious bronchitis

107 Acute tracheitis in a broiler. Secondary *E. coli* infection is established. Tracheal inflammation may vary from diffuse inflammation to a barely perceptible increase in production of a watery mucus. Gross lesions are occasionally confined to the bronchi and obstruction of these with inspissated inflammatory exudate may result in asphyxiation of the bird.

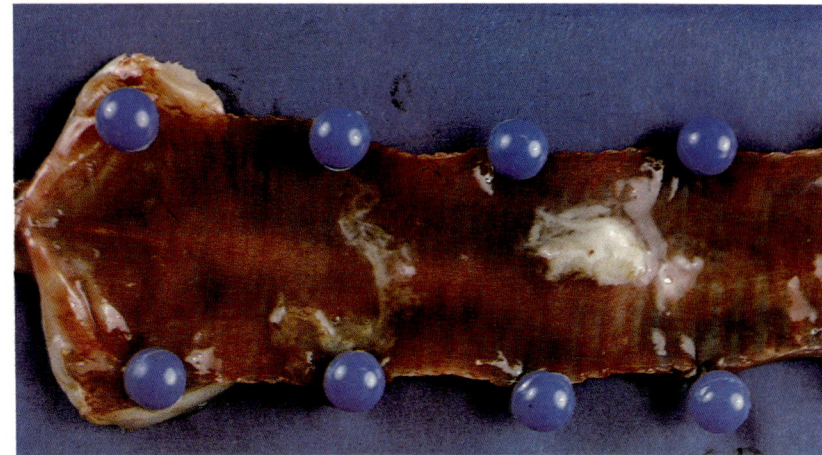

108 A dense lymphocytic infiltration is present in the tracheal mucosa of an unvaccinated 6-week-old broiler breeder. This type of lesion is often seen in field cases but is of doubtful specificity.

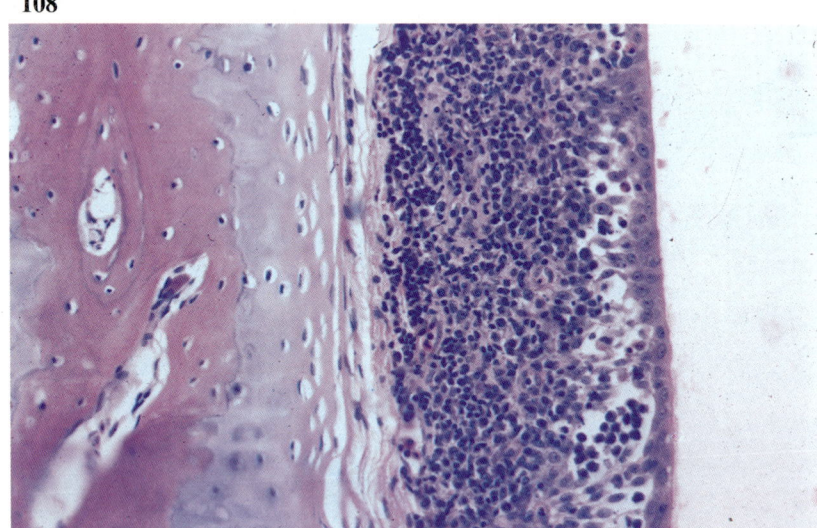

109 Acute nephritis in an unvaccinated 6-week-old broiler breeder. Infectious bronchitis virus was isolated from this tissue.

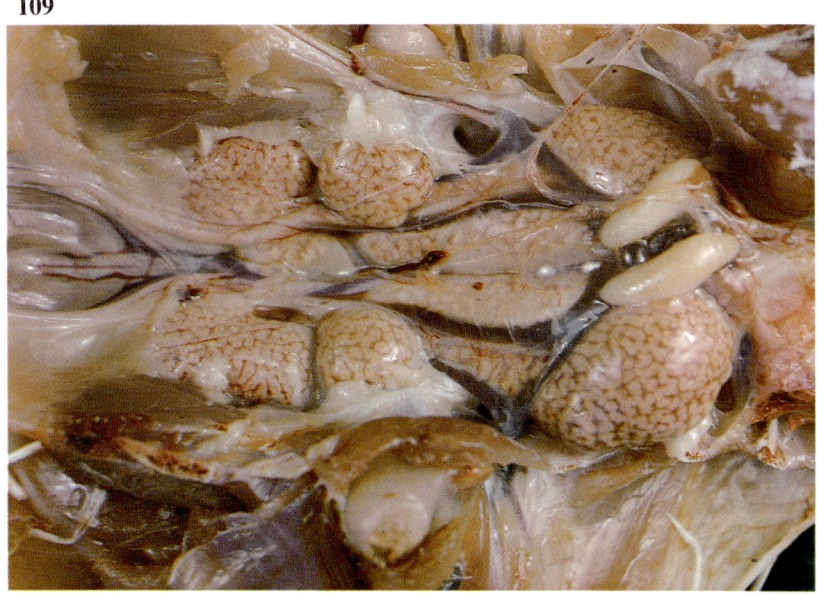

110 Interstitial nephritis produced in an experimental challenge of previously unvaccinated 10-week-old fowls with the H52 strain of the virus. This lesion was characterised by heavy mononuclear infiltration in which large numbers of plasma cells were present. Some plasma cells contain periodic acid schiff (PAS)-positive Russell bodies. PAS-haematoxylin.

110

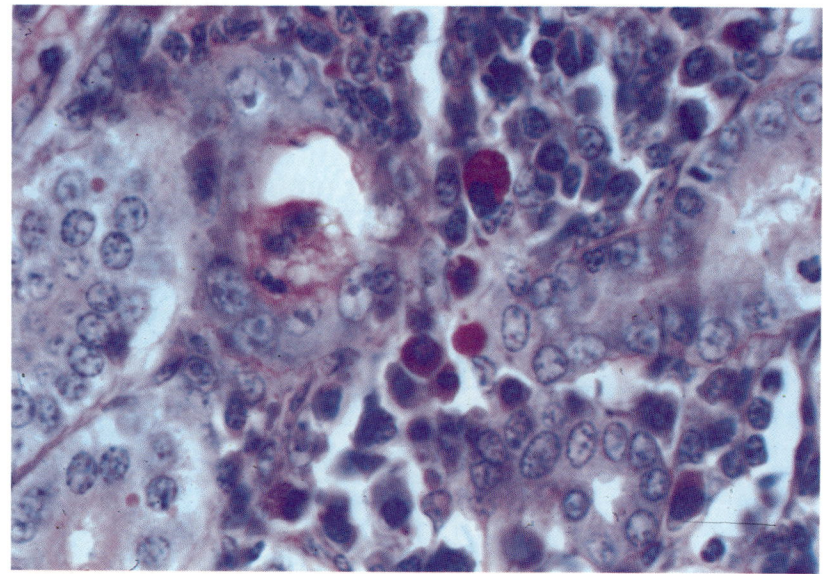

111 A wide range of egg abnormalities may be observed if susceptible laying fowl are infected. Shells are often ridged or have concretions on their surface. In others, as here, shells may be misshapen in other ways.

111

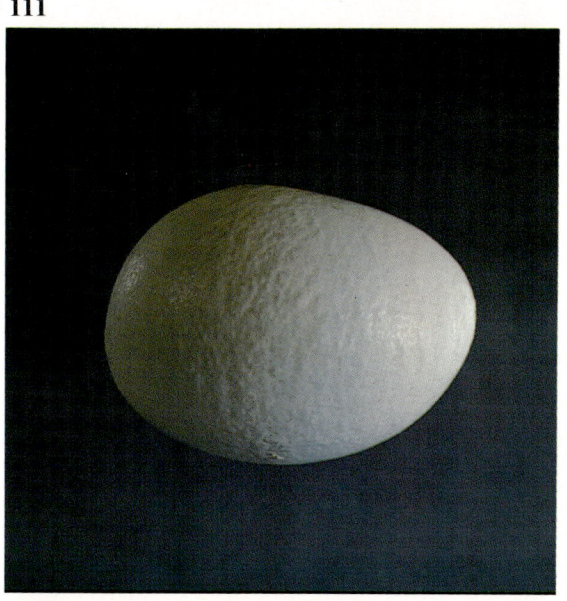

112 The internal quality of eggs may also suffer. In this photograph the light is being reflected from the outer rim of a watery egg white and there is no internal ring of albumen.

112

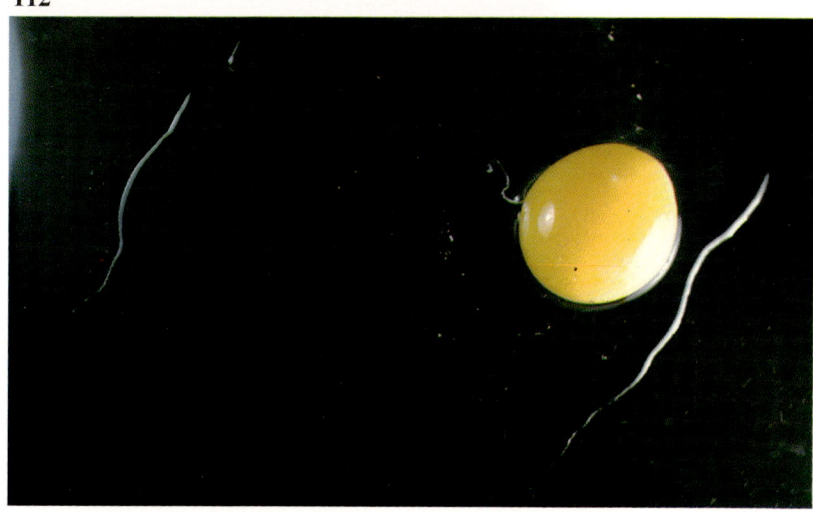

Egg drop syndrome '76
(127 adenovirus/BC14 infection)

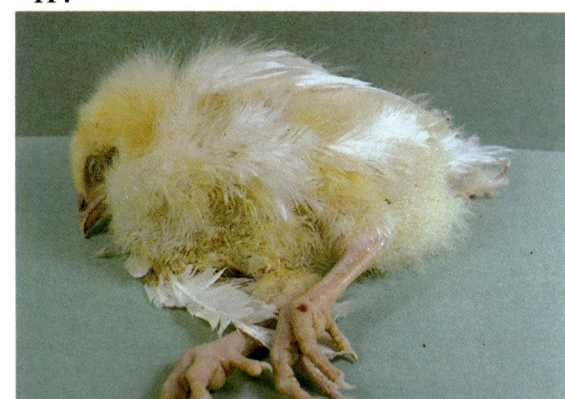

113 This infection is characterised by a drop in egg production or by a failure to peak in laying fowl. Both may be accompanied by the production of abnormally shelled eggs. These specimens are ridged, irregularly shaped and some have very thin shells. Soft-shelled and shell-less eggs may be seen.

Infectious avian encephalomyelitis
(epidemic tremor)

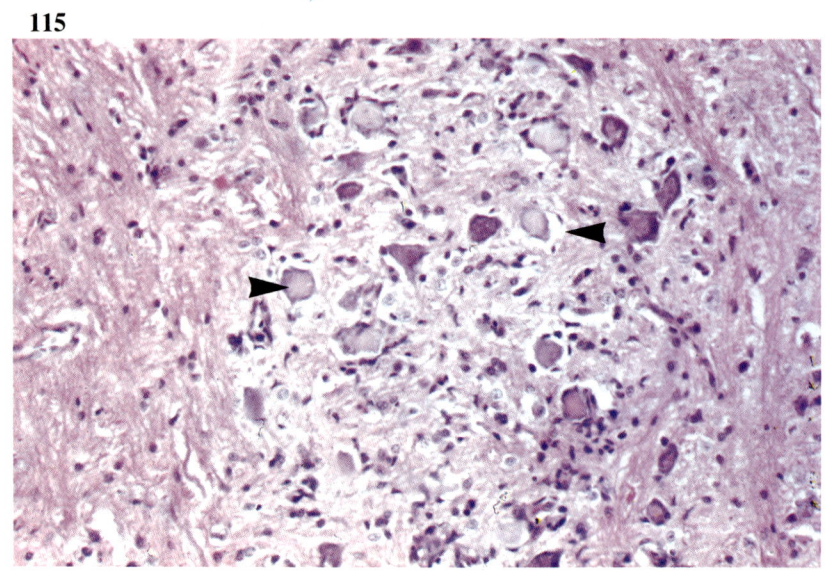

114 Terminal stages as in this 14-day-old chick may be preceded by ataxia. Muscular tremors may also be appreciated. Diagnosis is supported by histological examination of brain, spinal cord, pancreas, proventriculus, gizzard and heart. The disease occasionally occurs in turkeys.

115 A non-purulent encephalomyelitis is widely distributed throughout the spinal cord and brain. Degenerate neurons often exhibit central chromatolysis (arrows). This is not a pathognomonic feature but it can be a useful diagnostic sign as more neurons show degeneration of this type than in, say, either Marek's disease or Newcastle disease.

116 A brain stem neuron undergoing central chromatolysis. The nucleus has moved to the margin of the cell. Note the surrounding gliosis.

116

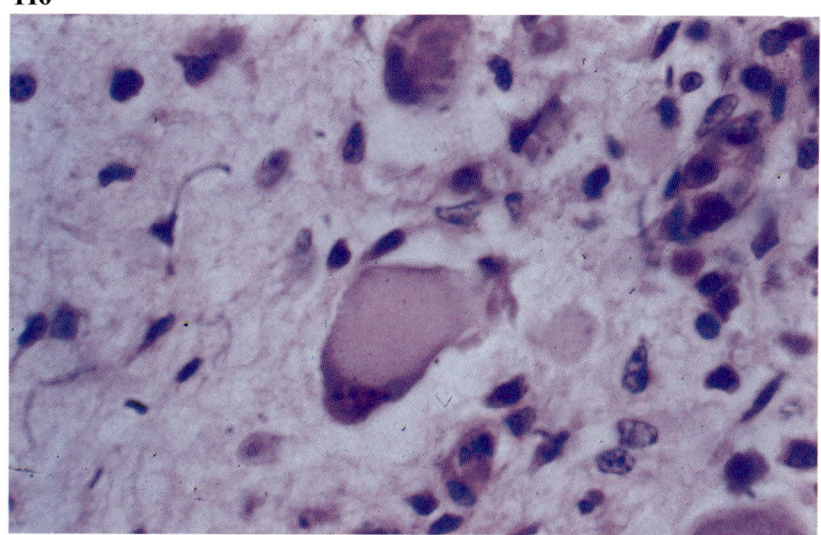

117 Visceral lesions are characterised by the presence of lymphoid infiltration. The pancreas normally contains a few lymphoid foci but in this section there is an increase in their number.

117

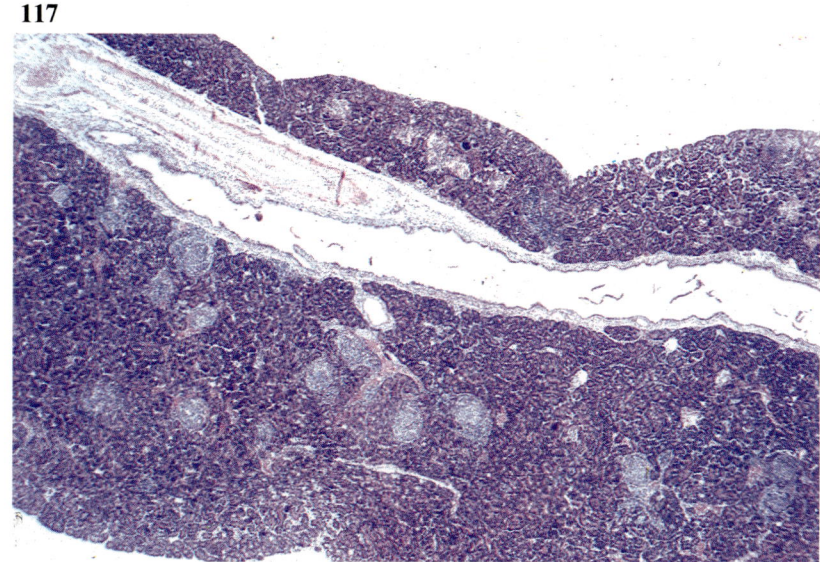

118 Higher power examination of one of the foci from **117** shows that it is mainly composed of immature cells.

118

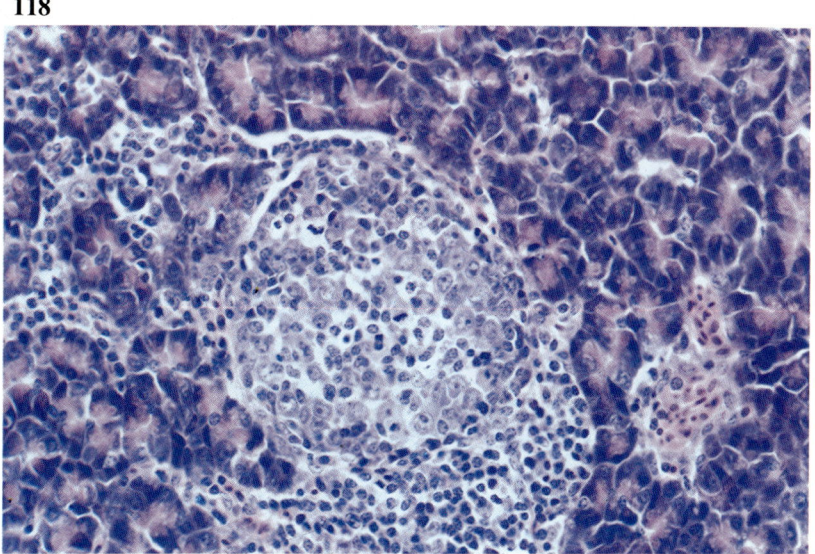

119 Lymphoid infiltration in the proventriculus is restricted to the muscularis. Similar infiltration may occur in the muscle of the gizzard and myocardium.

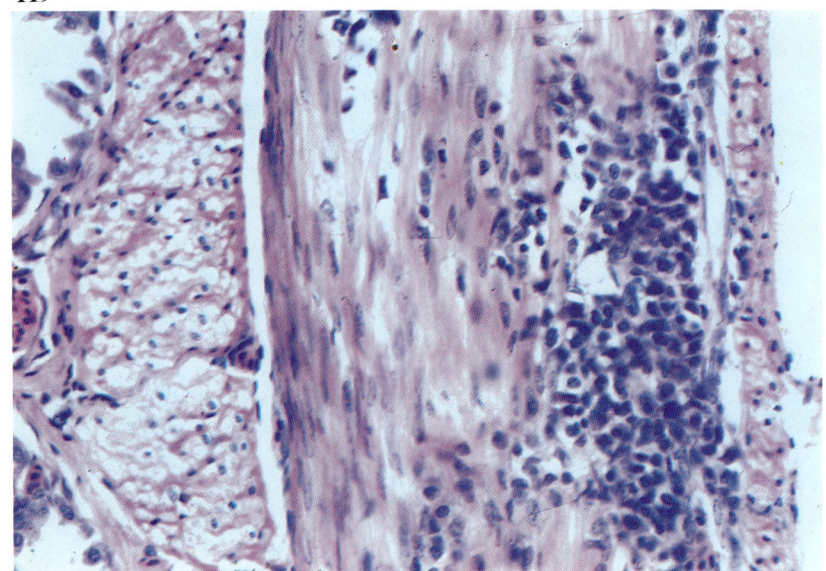

Viral arthritis and tenosynovitis

120 Ruptured gastrocnemius tendon as a result of chronic tendinitis in a broiler. Experimental reovirus infection (*see* **292**).

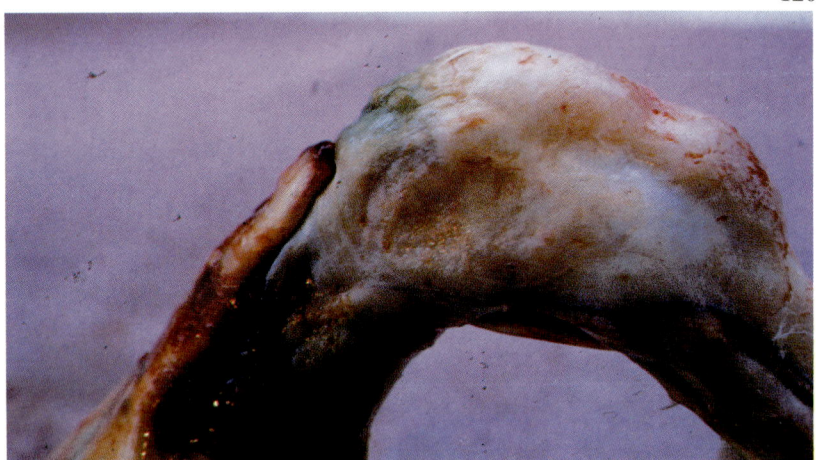

121 Ruptured digital flexor tendons in a broiler. Reovirus was isolated from this field case.

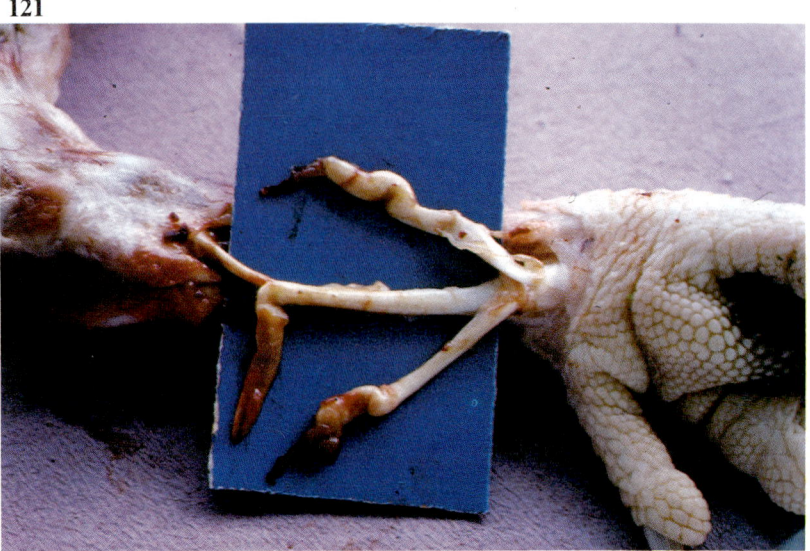

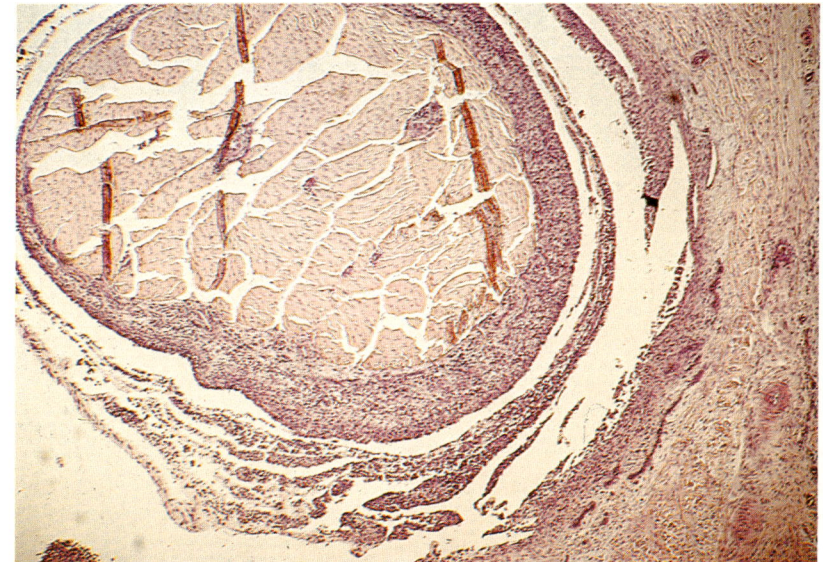

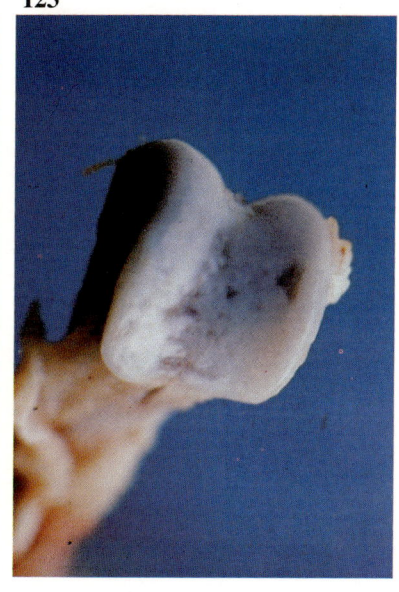

122 Tenosynovitis in a broiler. The tendon sheath is thickened as a result of a non-purulent inflammation involving a heavy infiltration of lymphocytes and plasma cells. Experimental reovirus infection.

123 Arthritic lesion with pitting of the articular cartilage over the distal tibiotarsal condyles in a broiler. Experimental reovirus infection. (*see* **30**).

Marek's disease (including transient paralysis)

124 Paresis of the right leg. If both legs are involved a characteristic posture is often taken up with one leg pointing forwards and the other held backwards under the body.

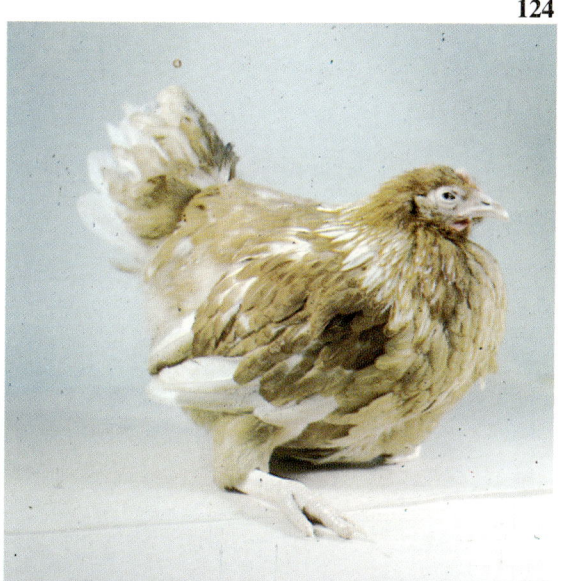

125 This normal sciatic nerve demonstrates the presence of cross striations. These are best seen in daylight rather than under artificial light and are gradually lost as post-mortem changes advance. In Marek's disease, if neural lesions are present, the first appreciable change is a loss of the normal striations together with some focal swelling and yellowing.

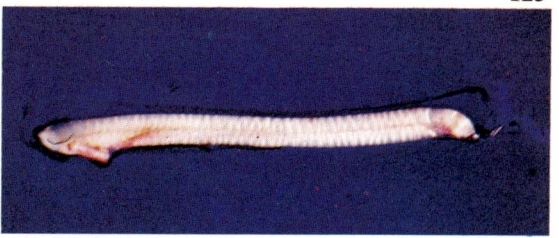

126 One brachial plexus is grossly enlarged. It is important to compare the vagal, brachial, intercostal, mesenteric and sciatic nerves both in the same bird and between individuals within a batch, otherwise slight swelling which may evenly affect most of the peripheral nerves can be missed. There is little doubt about the diagnosis of Marek's disease when gross neural lesions are found. Doubt arises when tumours are present in the organs in the absence of peripheral nerve enlargement. It is then necessary to examine both the nerves and neoplastic tissue histologically.

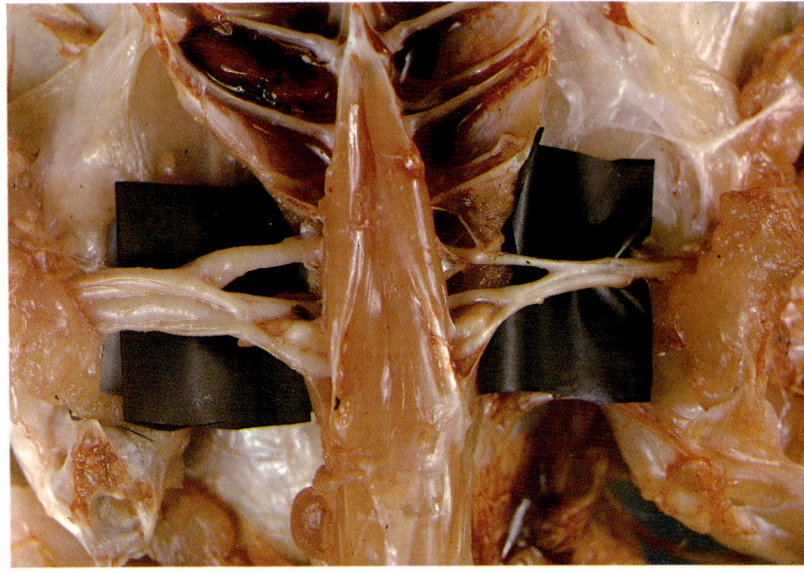

127 Small lymphocytes are aggregated around an intraneural capillary (type C lesion). A few plasma cells are often present in lesions of this type.

128 An infiltration of small lymphocytes and plasma cells in a peripheral nerve is accompanied by oedema (type B lesion).

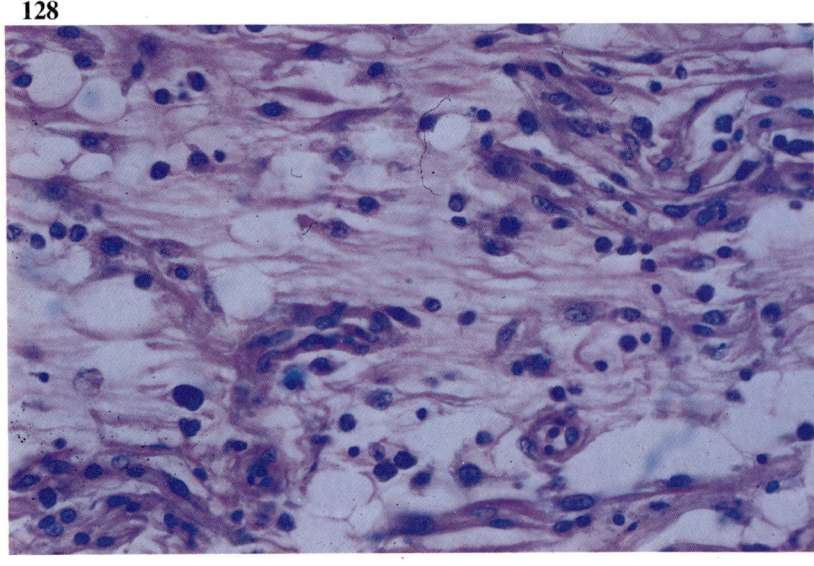

129 The tumorous spleen has ruptured and the subsequent haemorrhage caused the death of this 6-week-old broiler.

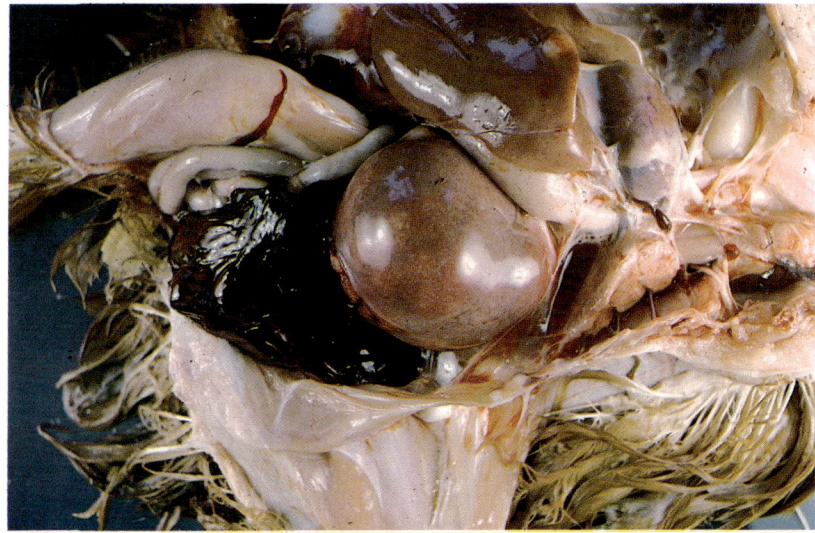

130 Tumour of wing muscle. Muscular and proventricular tumours occur more frequently in Marek's disease than in lymphoid leukosis.

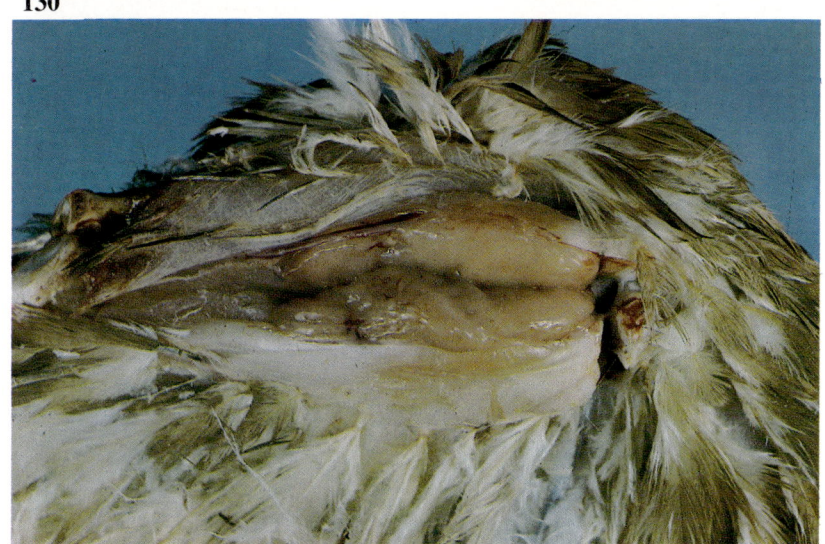

131 Grossly enlarged liver. Marek's disease tumours may involve most of the abdominal and thoracic viscera although the distribution varies considerably.

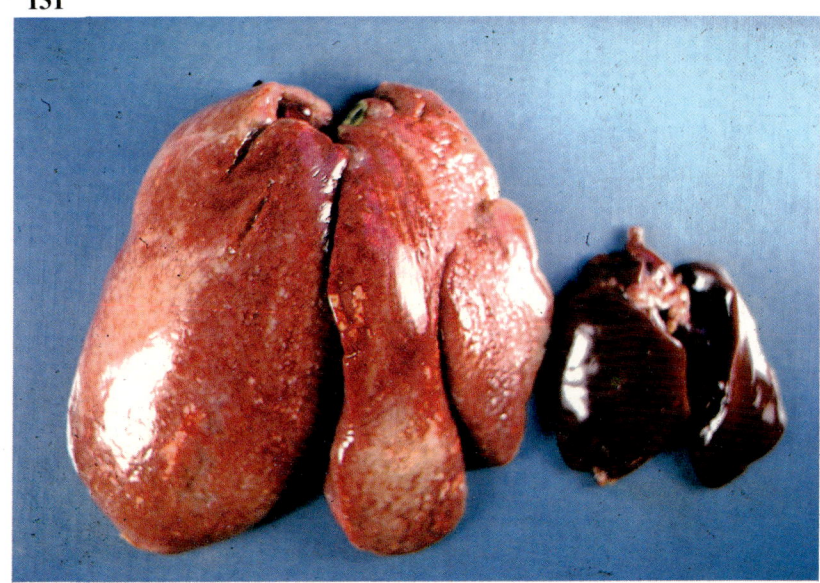

132 Skin tumours are uncommon in Britain but are sometimes encountered in broilers at slaughter. Most of the tumour formation in this specimen is taking place around the feather follicles.

132

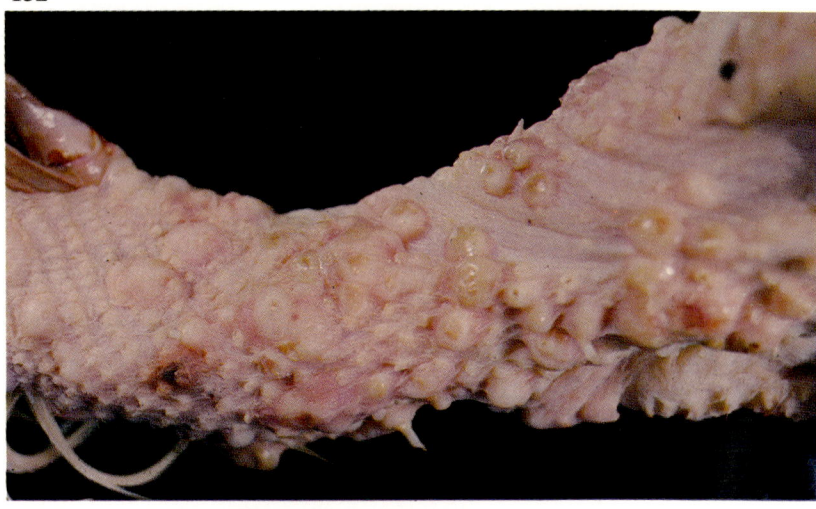

133 This small intestinal villus contains a laminal infiltrate of neoplastic lymphoid cells. The epithelium on the right is also parasitised with coccidial forms which are similar to those of *Eimeria acervulina*. Concurrent infection with coccidia is often observed in affected birds on deep litter.

133

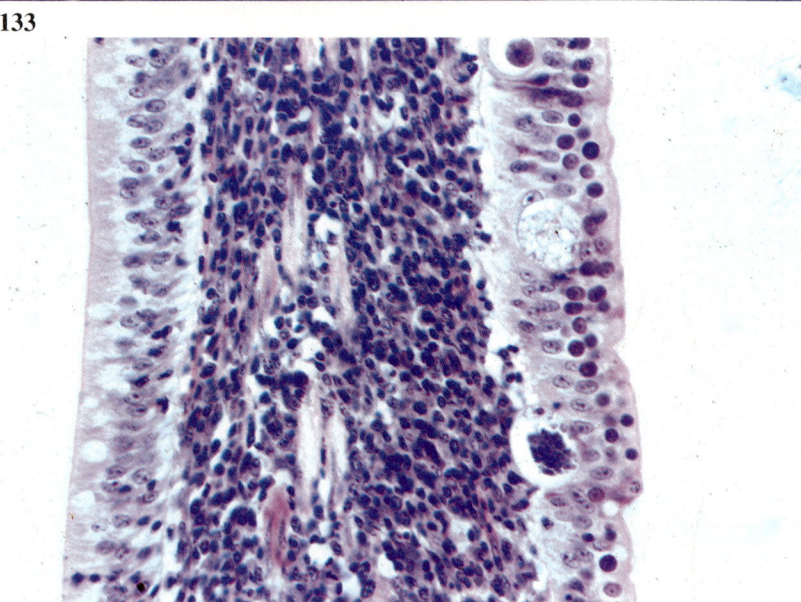

134 The population of neoplastic cells in Marek's disease tumours is nearly always pleomorphic. The section of skeletal muscle demonstrates this feature. A large dark staining cell is visible centrally, this is a so-called Marek's disease cell and is probably a degenerative lymphoblast. These cells are useful diagnostically but are relatively infrequent. *NB* The type A lesion of peripheral nerve is also composed of proliferating mixed lymphoid cells.

134

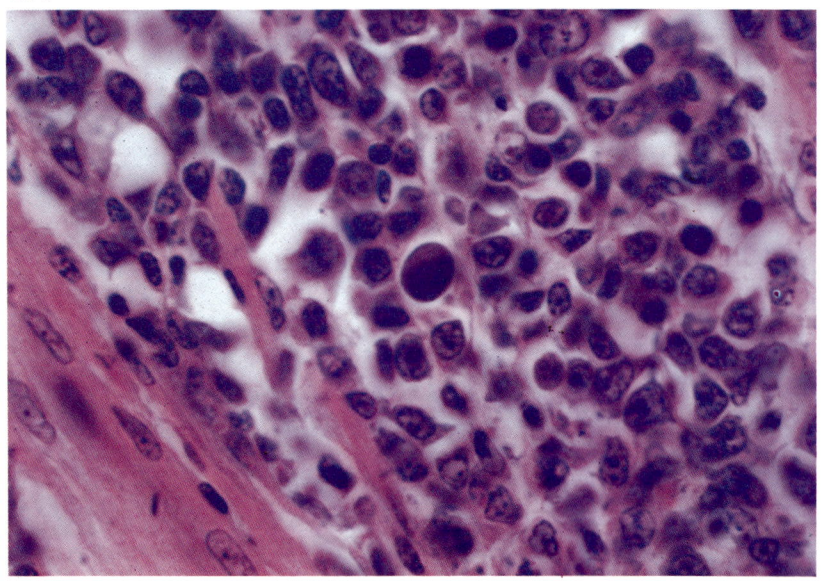

135 The cut surface of this liver demonstrates grey areas of lymphoid infiltration round the portal triads and central veins. This type of infiltration is frequently seen in Marek's disease.

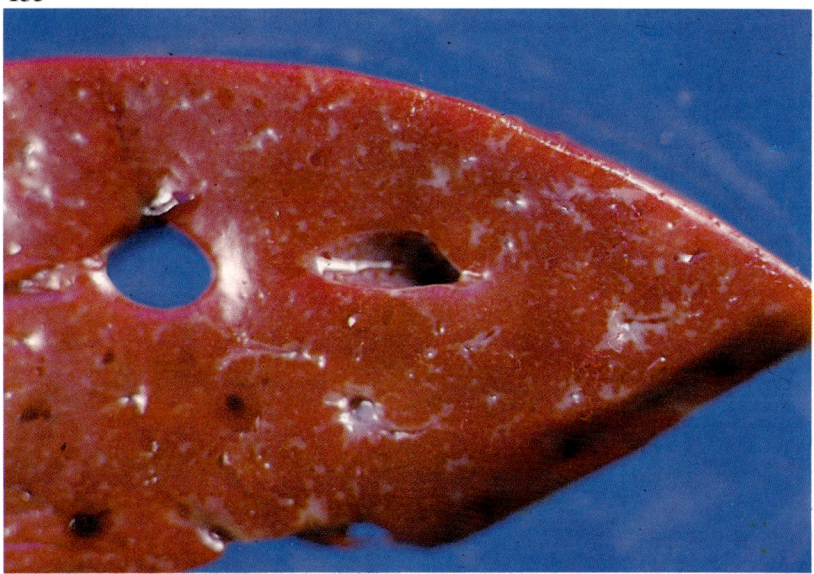

136 This section of an autolysing visceral tumour demonstrates numerous pyknotic nuclei within degenerating neoplastic lymphoid cells. Pyknosis tends to be seen more frequently in autolysing lesions of Marek's disease than in those of lymphoid leukosis (*see* **146**).

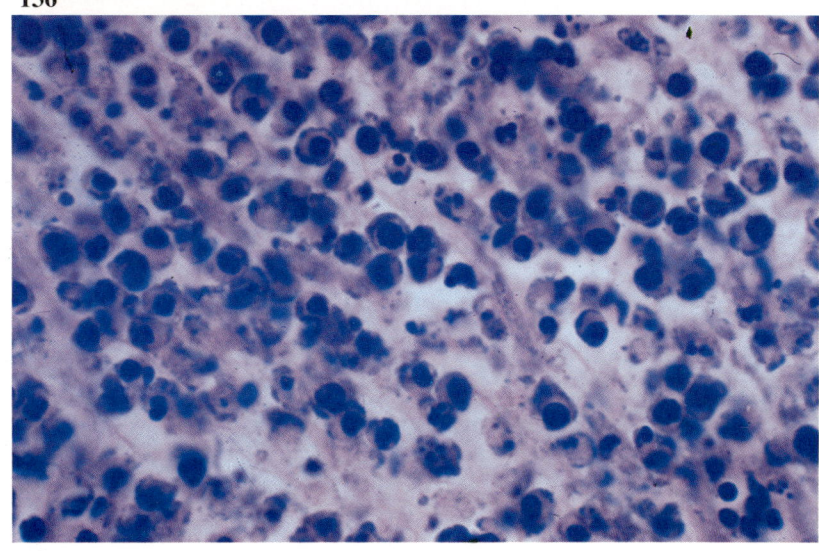

137 Dense perivascular cuffing is a feature of an encephalitis which affects some birds.

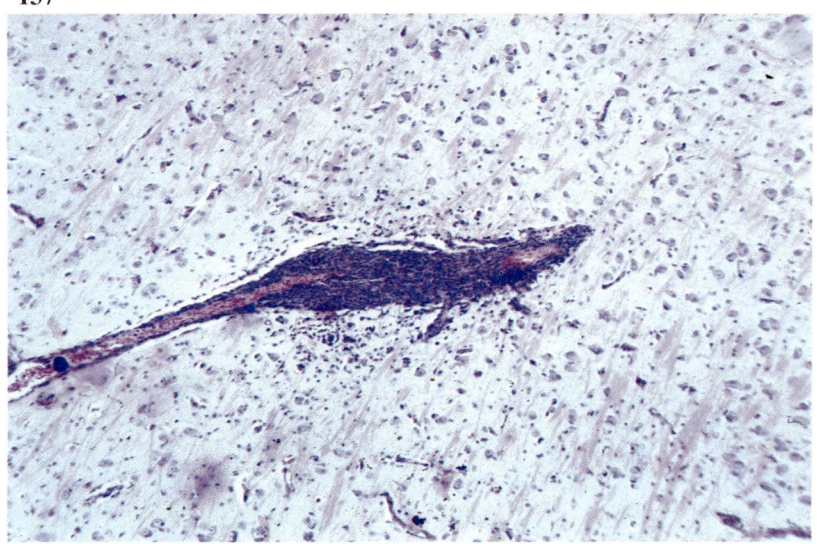

138 Transient paralysis. This pullet shows flaccid paralysis of the neck and tail.

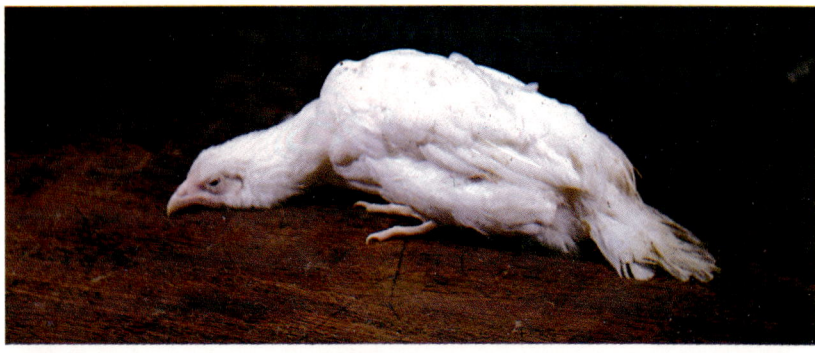

139 A perivascular cuff in the brain of a bird showing signs of transient paralysis. Note the small cyst-like foci of nuclear debris (arrows).

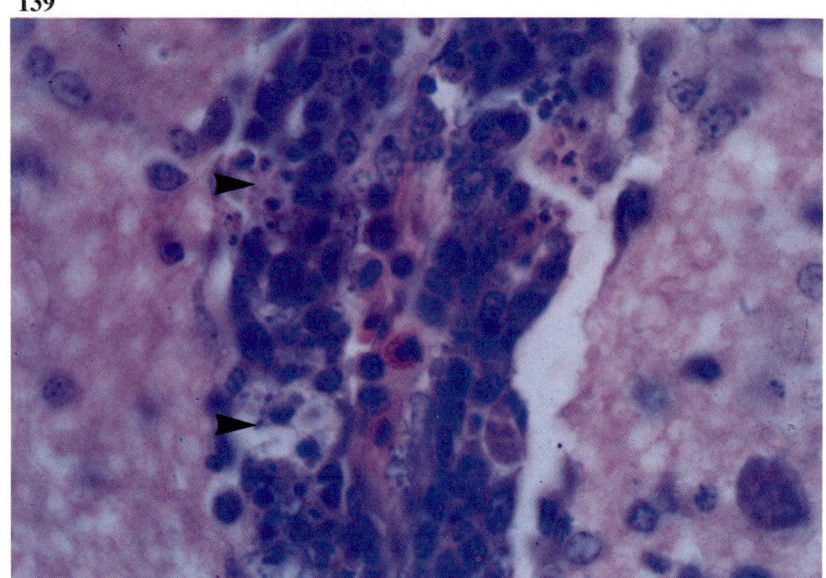

Lymphoid leukosis and other tumours caused by the leukosis/sarcoma group of viruses

140 The liver of this adult fowl is greatly enlarged due to extensive neoplastic infiltration. In the past this condition was often called 'big liver disease'. Although hepatic tumours are often found, the macroscopic appearance of the liver cannot be relied on for diagnosis.

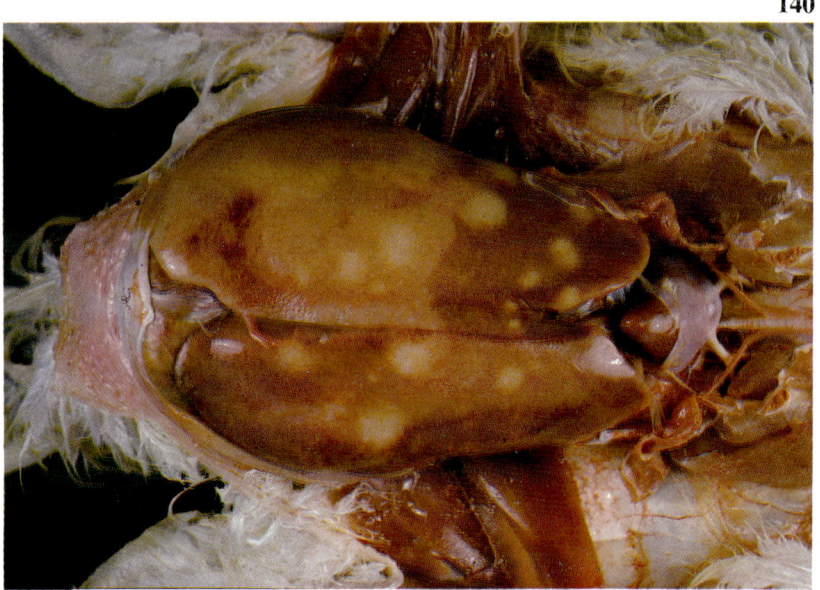

141 Lymphoid tumours affecting the kidneys and bursa of Fabricius in the same bird depicted in **140**.

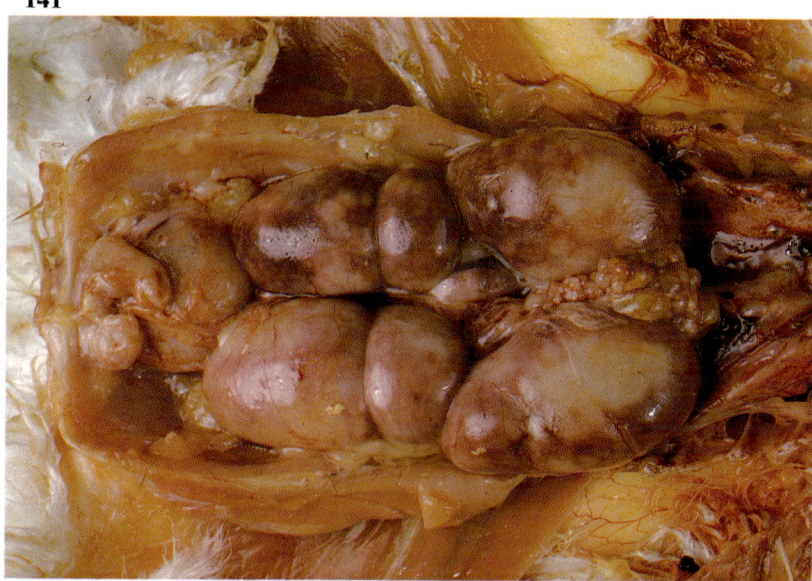

142 Tumour formation causing great enlargement of the bursa of Fabricius and focal hepatic lesions in an adult fowl.

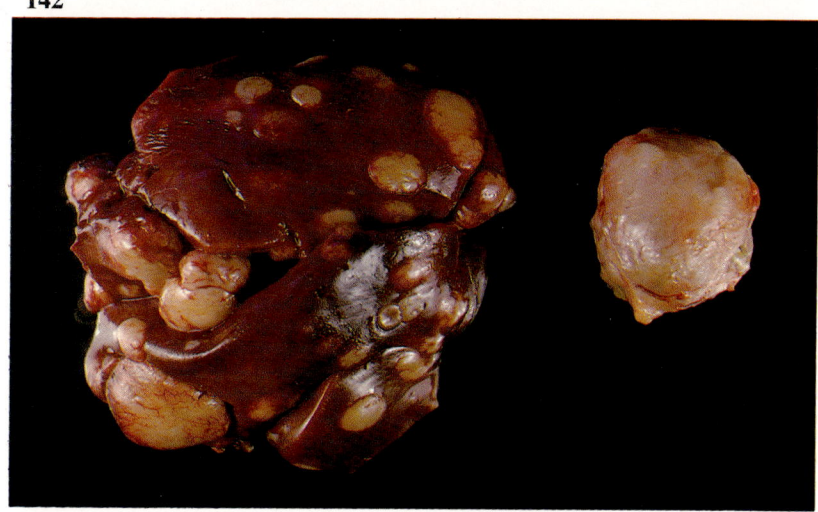

143 Tumours are focal and grow by expansion. This contrasts with the more infiltrative lesions of Marek's disease. Cords of hepatocytes are being compressed between expanding foci in this liver.

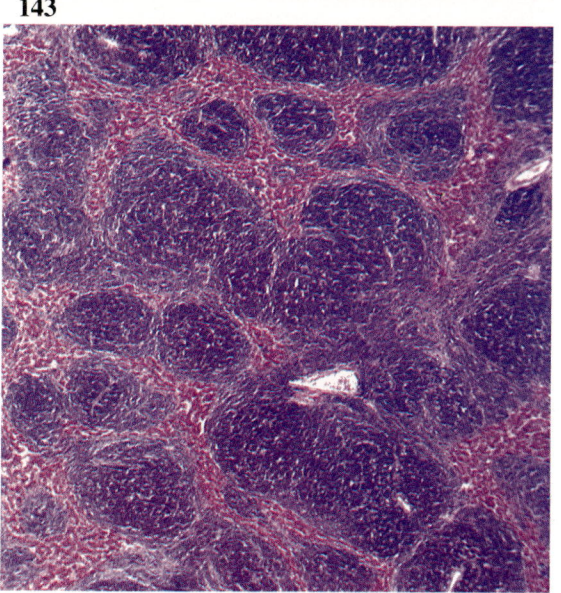

144 Expansion of the primary intra-follicular tumours taking place in the bursa of Fabricius.

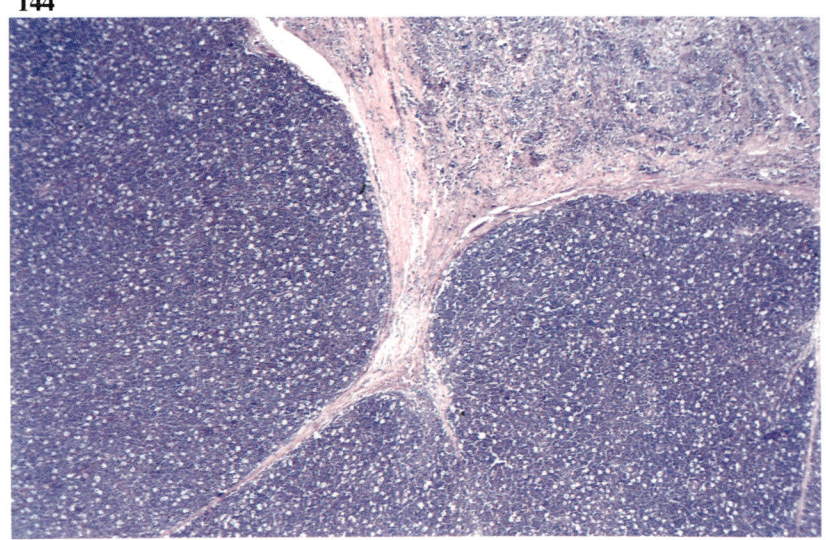

145 Tumours are composed of sheets of immature cells which show little or no pleomorphism. Frequently, the nuclei are surrounded by a clearly defined rim of cytoplasm and contain large violet-staining nucleoli.

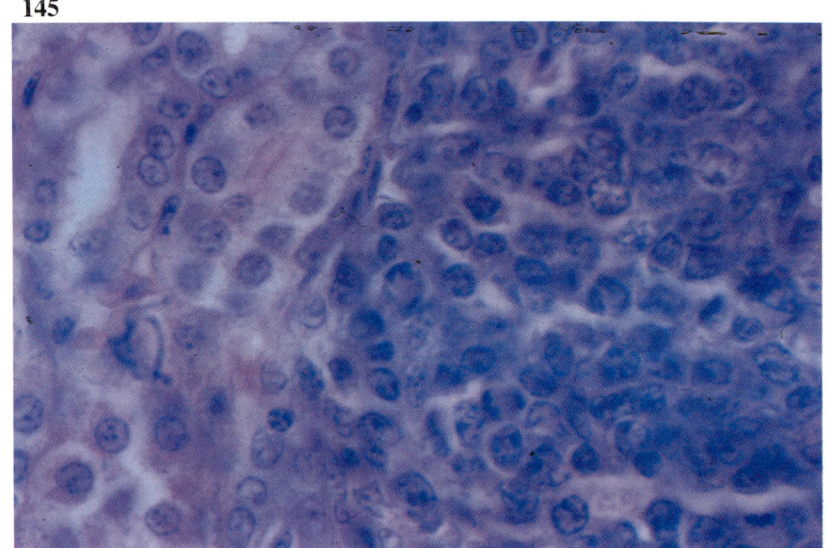

146 Many of the tumour cell nuclei undergo karyorrhexis during auto-lysis (*see* **136**).

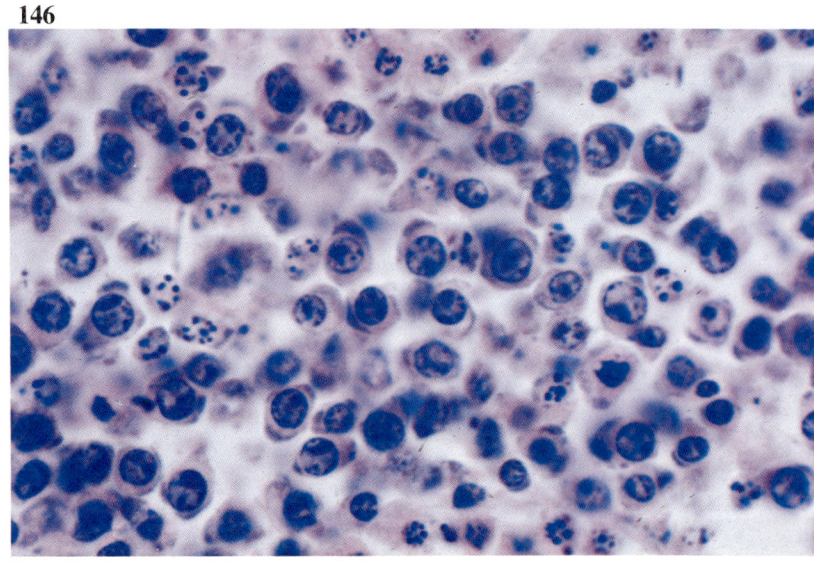

147 Myeloid leukosis. Chalky white myelocytomas are present on the sternum and ribs of this fowl.

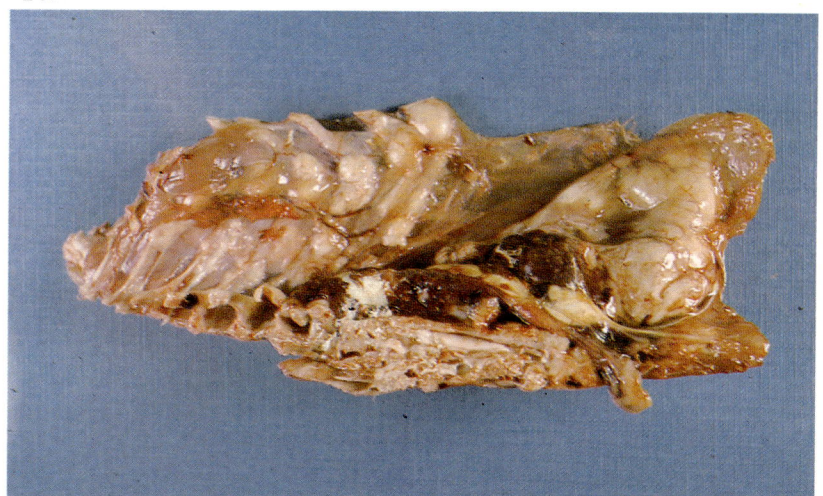

148 Myeloid leukosis. Large numbers of proliferating myelocytes infiltrating skeletal muscle.

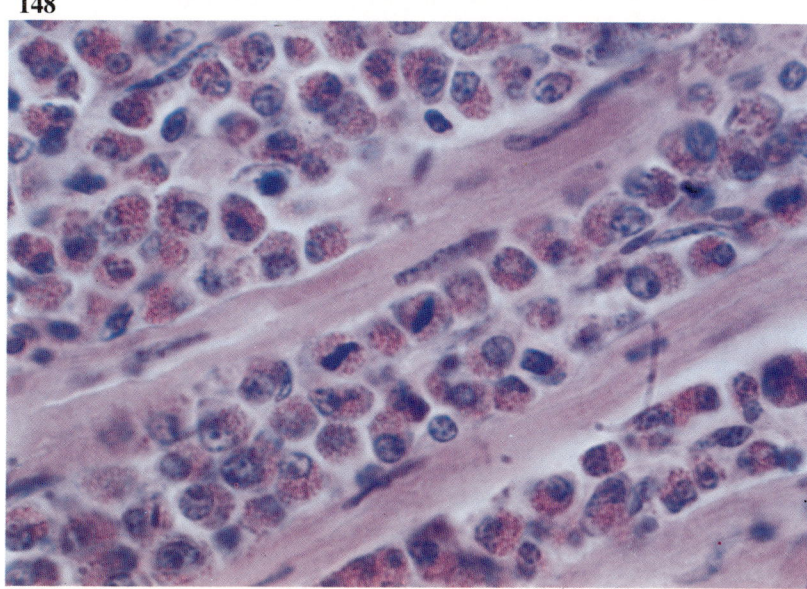

149 Erythroid leukosis. The liver of this fowl is greatly enlarged and cherry red. Similar lesions may occur in the spleen. The condition is rare.

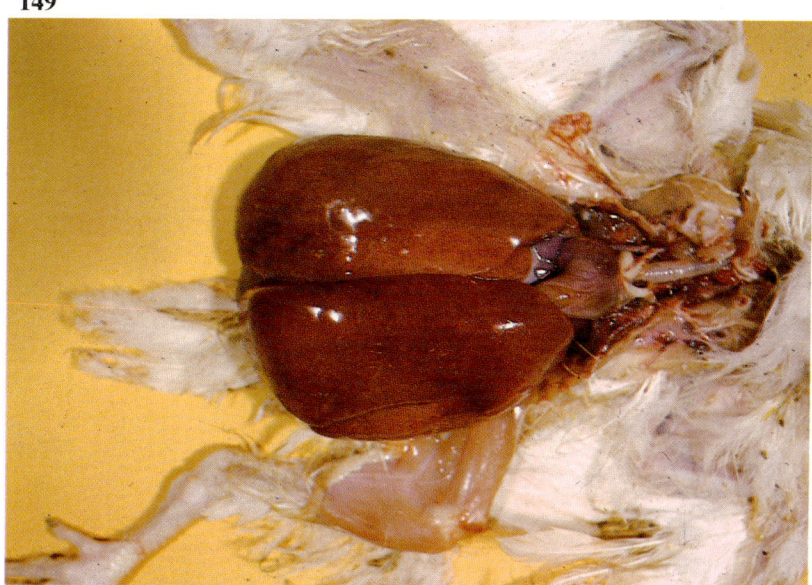

150 Osteopetrosis. Cross section of an affected tarsometatarsus in a fowl shows the great increase in thickness of the cortical bone.

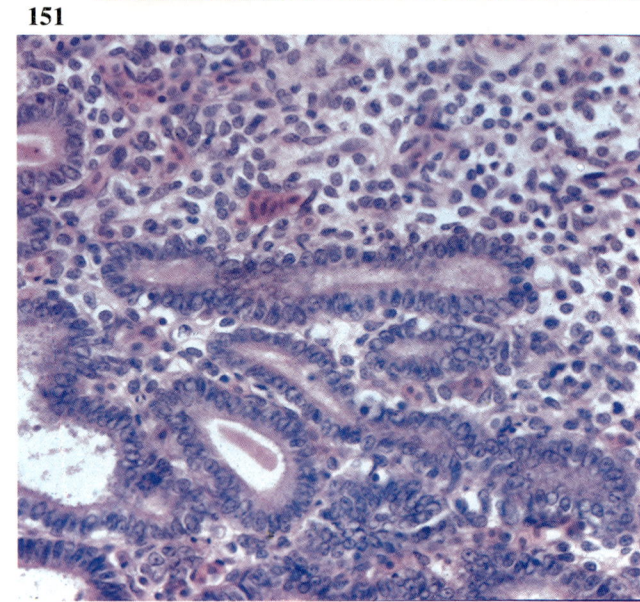

150

151 Nephroblastoma. This may be encountered in some fowl as a large tumour that has replaced a division of the kidney. They may be cystic. Histologically they are very variable. In this section tubular structures are surrounded by masses of undifferentiated cells.

151

152 Nephroblastoma. Keratinised forms of nephroblastoma are seen from time to time. Large whorls of keratin in this lesion are surrounded by a rim of epithelial cells.

152

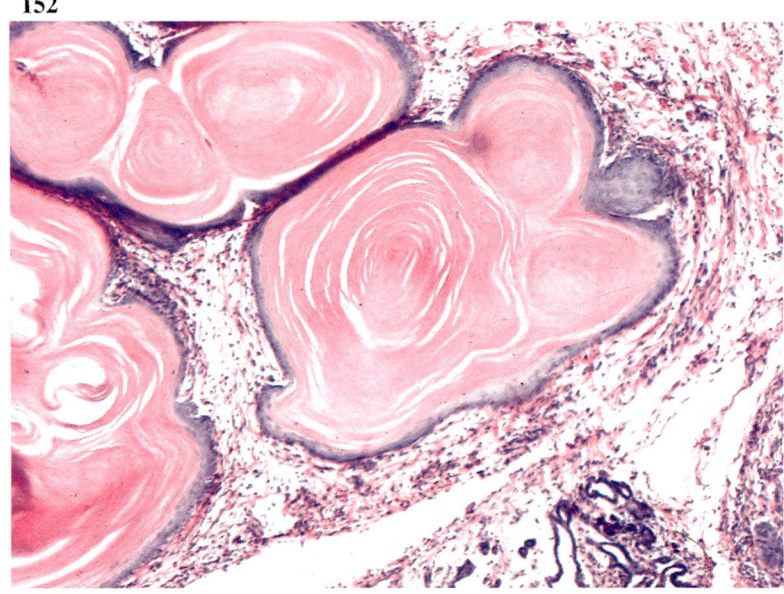

Lymphoproliferative disease of turkeys

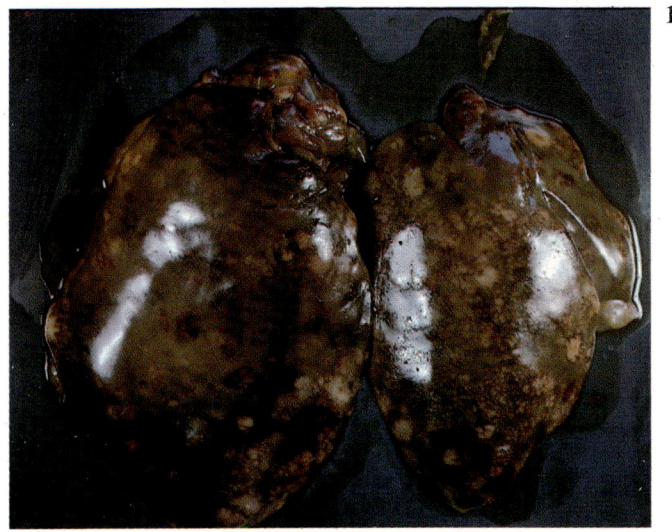

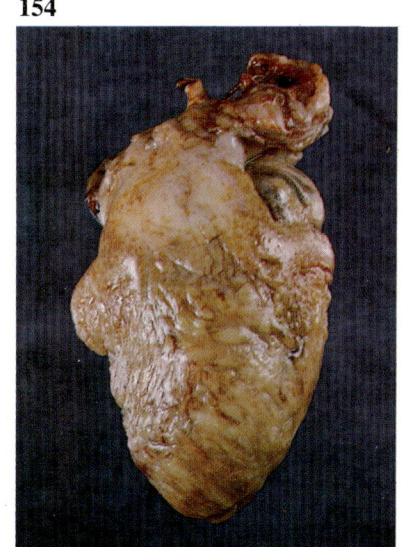

153 Greatly enlarged liver in a 15-week-old grower. This bird also had a *Pseudomonas aeruginosa* septicaemia. The spleen is often very enlarged in this condition.

154 Diffuse tumour of heart.

155 Section of liver showing the pleomorphic nature of the lymphoid tumour.

156 The lesion in **155** seen at higher magnification.

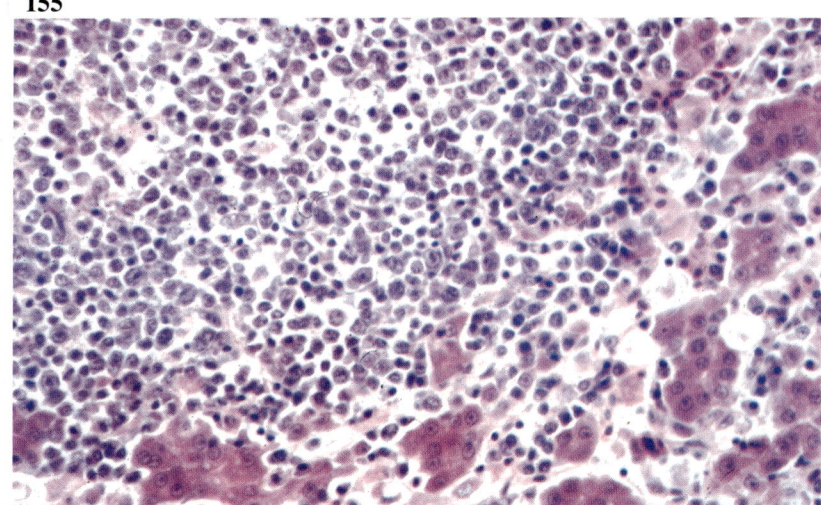

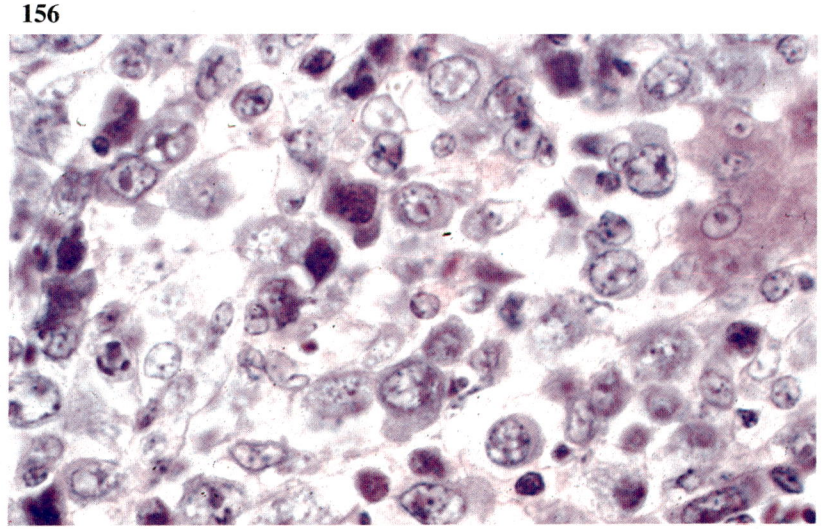

Reticuloendotheliosis virus induced tumours in turkeys

157 Experimental infection. The lesions are focal and grow by expansion. This section demonstrates the population of primitive lymphoblasts.

157

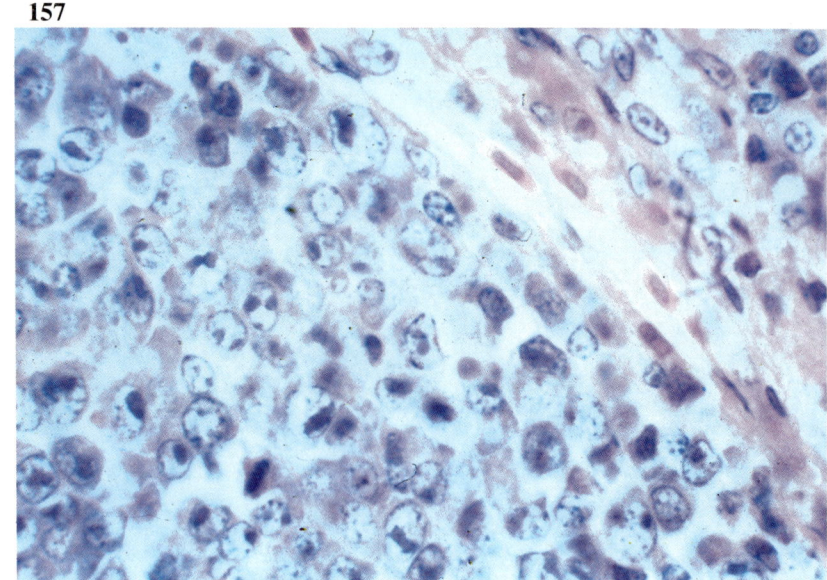

Other neoplasias

Adenocarcinoma of the reproductive tract of the hen

158 Carcinomas may arise from either the ovary or the oviduct. In this specimen the oviduct is principally involved but primary ovarian lesions are also common. The tumour tissue is pale and very firm on palpation. Lesions are seen towards the end of lay as a sporadic cause of death but occasional outbreaks occur.

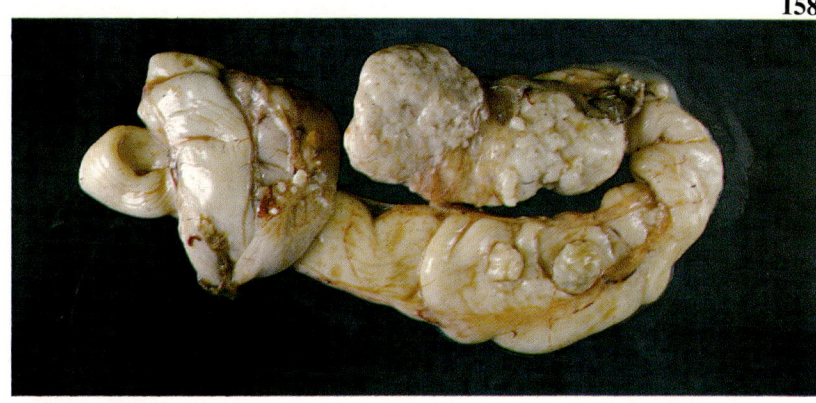
158

159 These tumours usually metastasise to serous surfaces in the abdominal cavity and particularly affect the pancreas, intestine and its mesentery. The metastatic nodules on the viscera are frequently rounded.

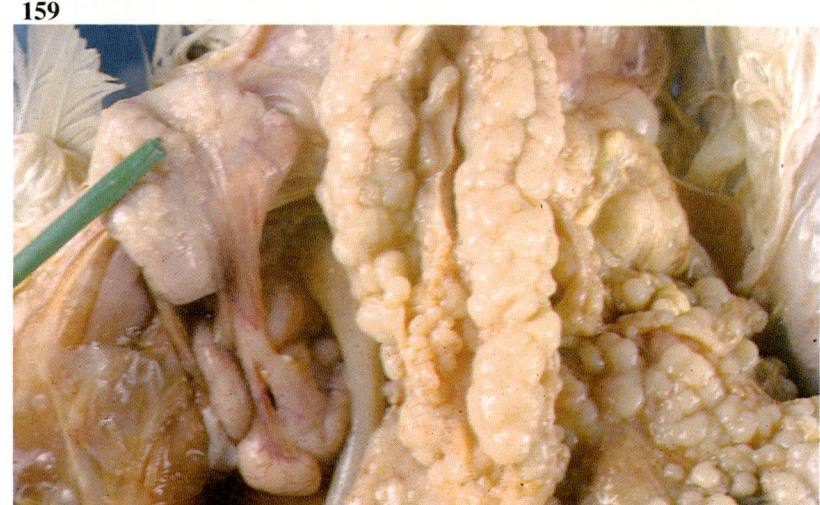
159

160 Most of the metastases are scirrhous in nature due to the proliferation of connective tissue in response to the invading carcinomatous cells.

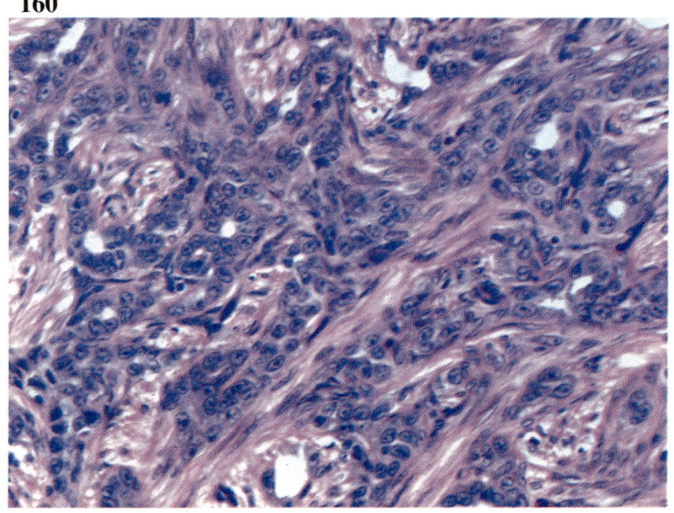
160

Leiomyoma of the oviduct ligaments

161 These tumours (arrow) are often found in the ventral ligament and are usually composed of both smooth muscle and fibrous elements.

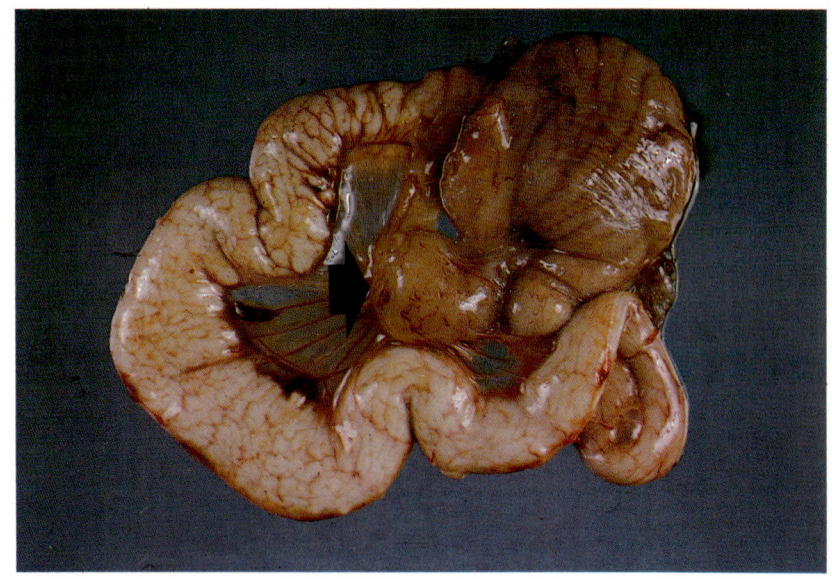

Squamous cell carcinoma of the skin

162 Multiple small crater-like lesions are occasionally found on inspection of broiler carcases at slaughter. Individual ulcers may coalesce, particularly on the back.

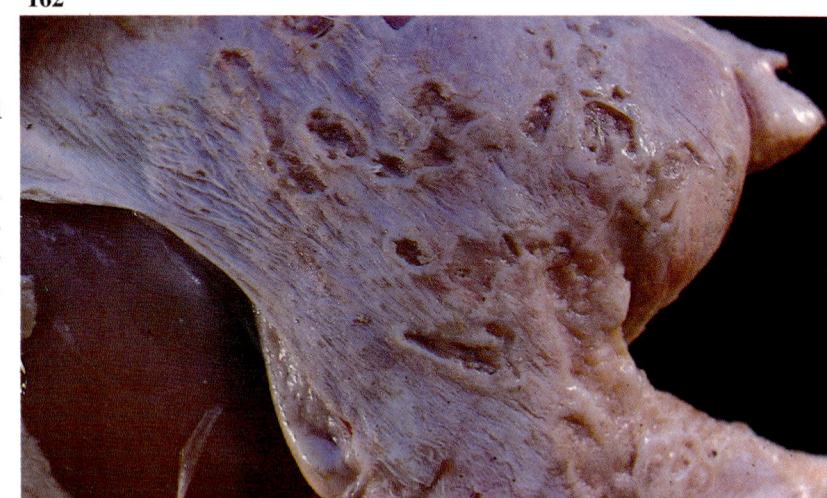
162

163 A keratin 'pearl' surrounded by squamous cells. The tumours invade the dermis and subcutaneous tissue but do not seem to metastasise during the commercial life of the broiler.

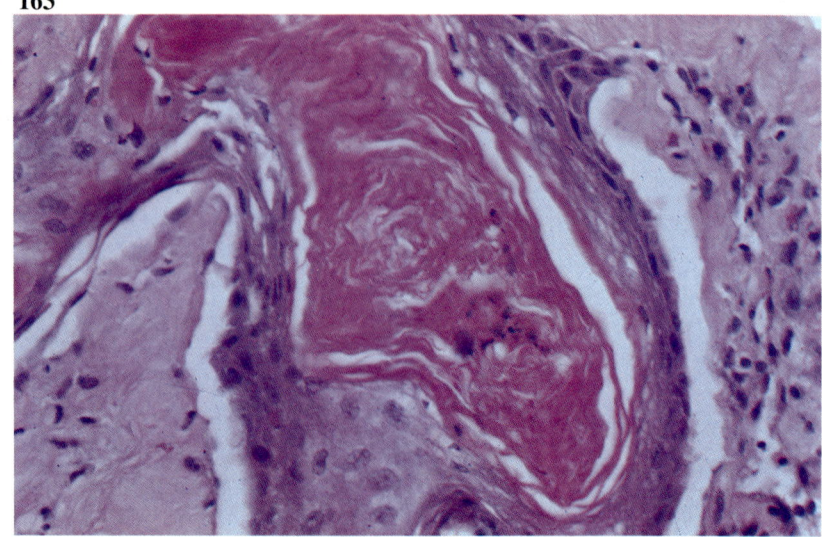
163

Fungal diseases

Aspergillosis

164 Miliary lesions of pneumonia caused by *A. fumigatus* in a 7-day-old chick that had been infected from contaminated straw litter. If infection is acquired in the hatchery – a rare event these days – pneumonia can develop by 2 days of age. Occasionally, lesions are confined to the bronchi and are not seen unless the lung is cut through.

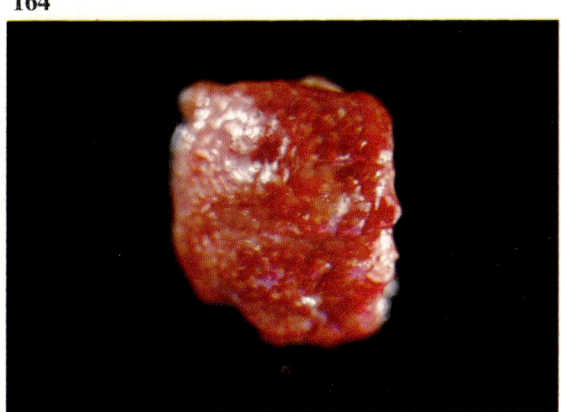

165 The miliary lesions in the lungs consist of rapidly developing granulomas. PAS-haematoxylin.

166 Necrotic tissue is quickly removed by giant cell activity. In this section hyphae are protruding through a ring of giant cells PAS-haematoxylin.

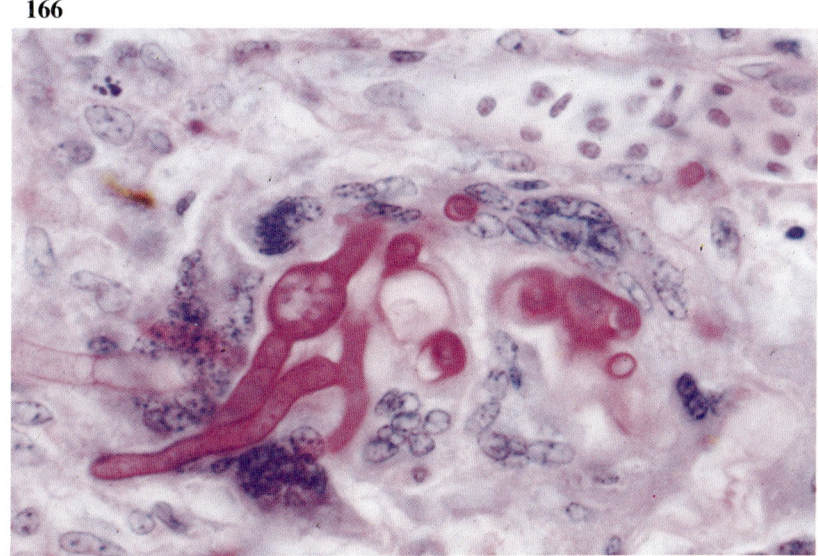

167 Infections in chicks and turkey poults often result in the development of small nodules on the surface of the thoracic and abdominal air sacs. These lesions have a concentric appearance and a depressed centre. Later growing stages in the turkey may be affected by an air sacculitis in which there are much larger plaques of pus present.

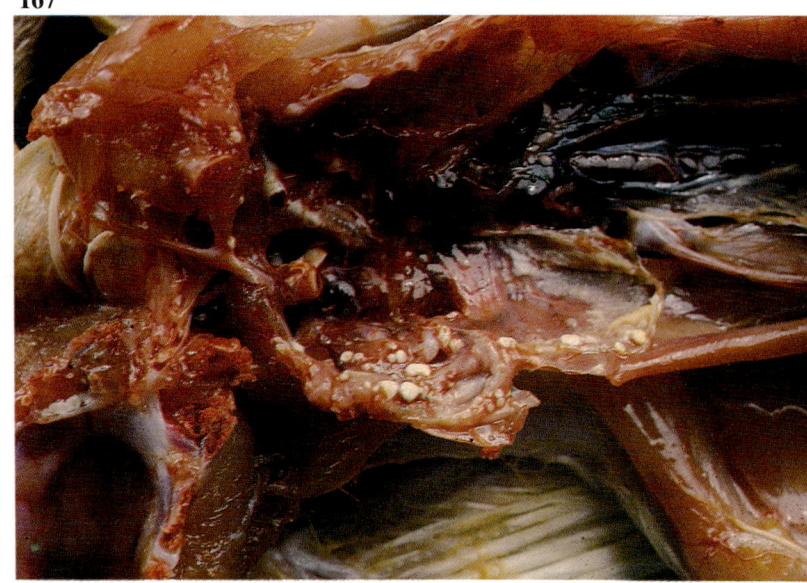

168 Heavy pulmonary infections in young birds may lead to focal encephalitis. Small hyphae in the brain stem of a turkey poult are surrounded by an intense inflammatory reaction and some attempt at early giant cell formation. PAS-haematoxylin.

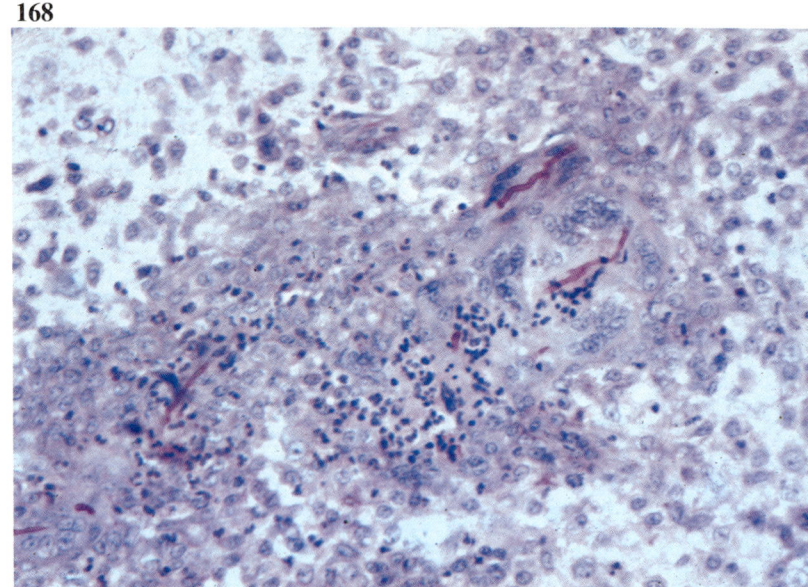

169 Conidiophores are sometimes seen if pulmonary lesions extend into an air space.

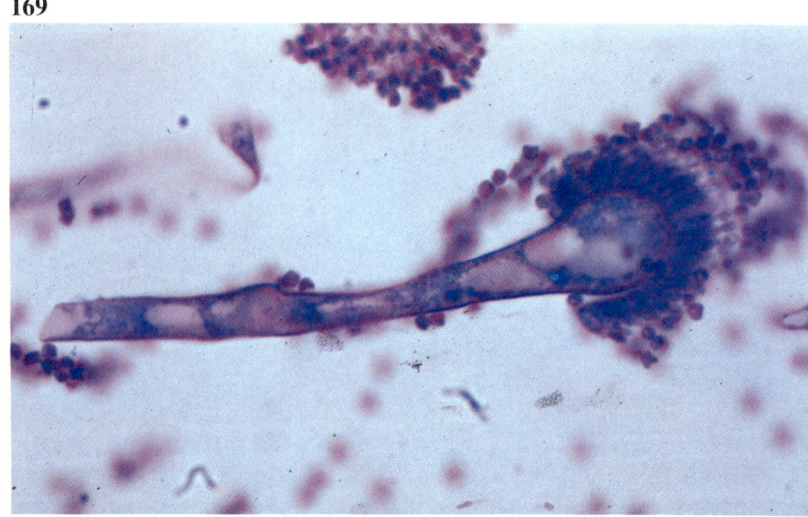

Dactylariosis

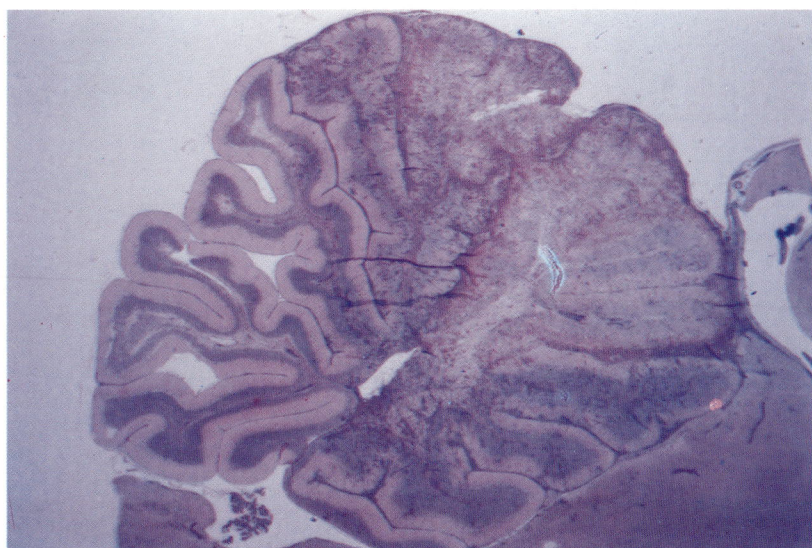

170 Occasional outbreaks may result in severe losses in both chicks and poults. *Dactylaria gallopava*, introduced as a contaminant on bark litter, caused heavy mortality in broilers on the farm from which this specimen was obtained. Pulmonary lesions were minimal but severe cerebellar and brain stem lesions caused an outbreak of disease which clinically resembled encephalomalacia. The infection has destroyed most of the posterior folia. PAS-haematoxylin.

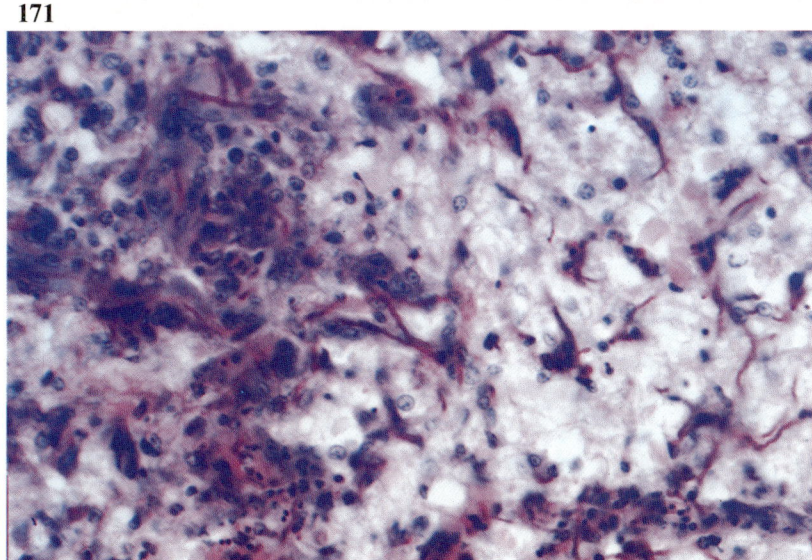

171 Higher magnification of **170** shows slender hyphae ensheathed by newly formed giant cells. PAS-haematoxylin.

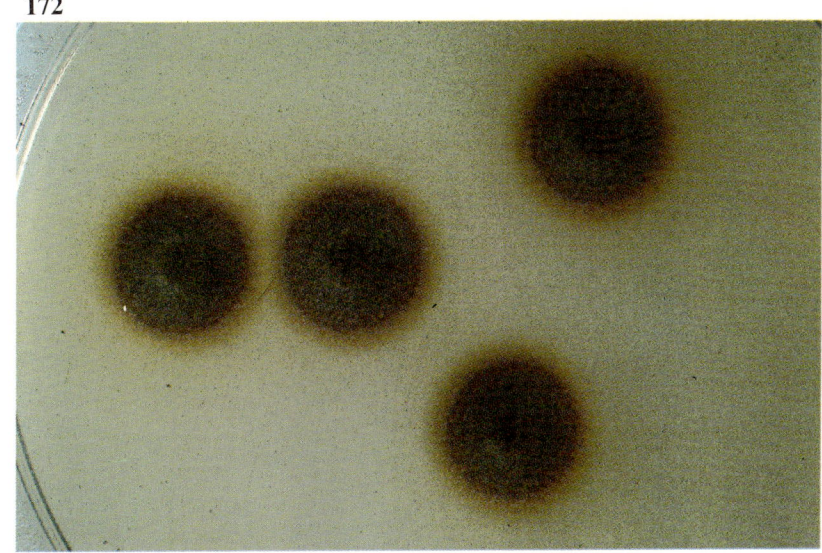

172 Young colonies of *D. gallopava* growing on Sabouraud's medium after 48 hours growth at 42°C.

Candidiasis

173 A heavy deposit of desquamated epithelial cells provides the typical 'turkish towelling' appearance. *Candida albicans* infection.

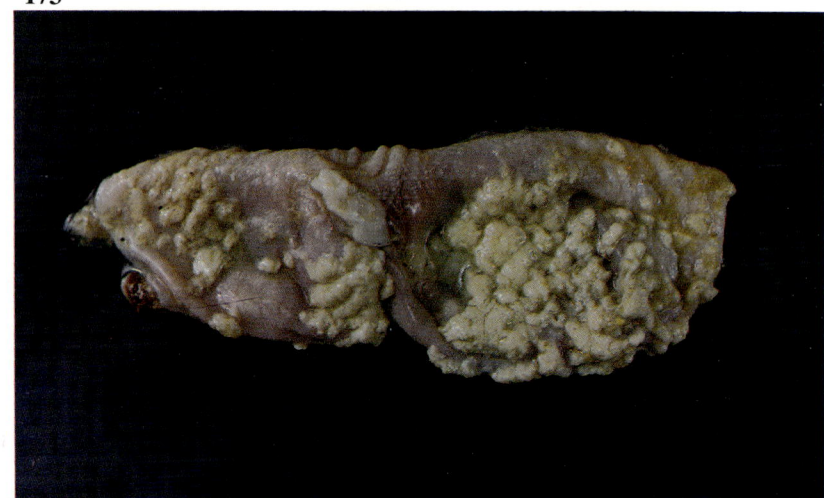

174 Most of the fungal growth takes place in the mass of degenerate squames but some invasion of the intact epithelium usually occurs. The pseudohyphae are poorly demonstrated with haematoxylin and eosin but are strongly positive to PAS and other fungal stains. PAS-haematoxylin.

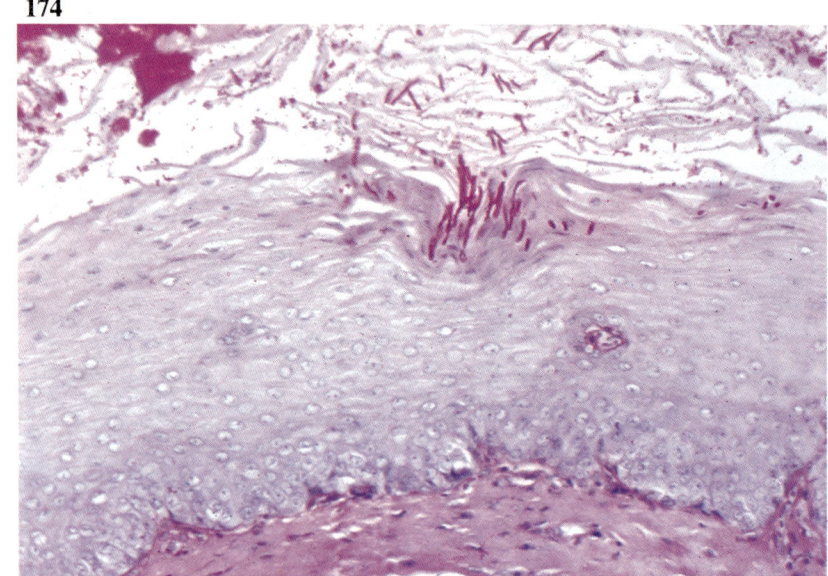

175 Pseudo-hyphae within crop epithelium. PAS-haematoxylin.

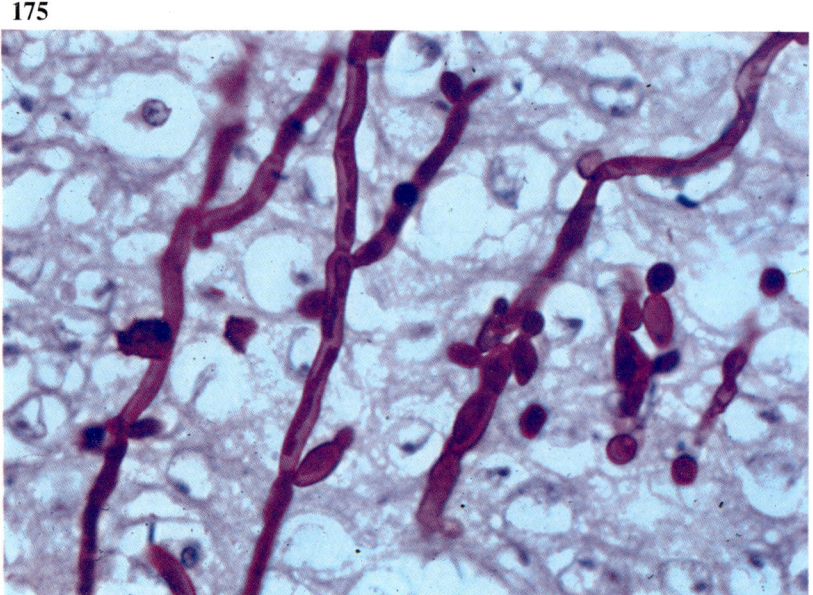

Parasitic diseases

Ascaridiasis

176 Heavy infestations with *Ascaridia galli* are not common under intensive systems of husbandry. Intercurrent disease such as Marek's disease may be present.

176

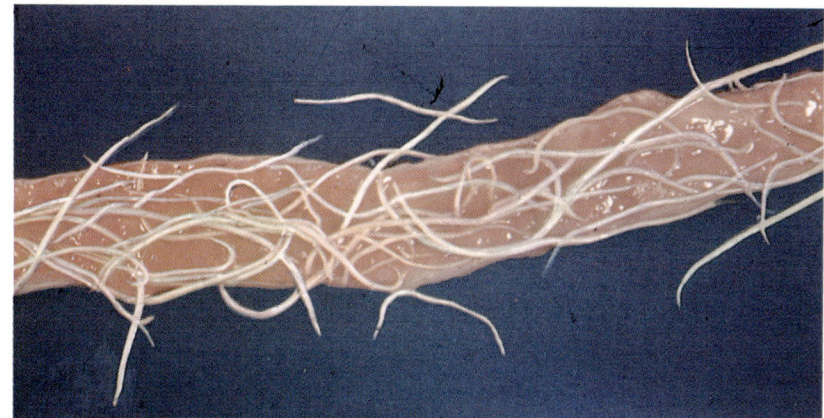

Capillariasis

177 Infestation of the small intestine may have a marked effect on egg production in fowls maintained on deep litter. The affected bowel is usually pale and distended with fluid contents; the mucosa is slightly roughened. The worms are difficult to see with the naked eye but are easily visible in smears. This photograph demonstrates the bi-operculate eggs within a female worm.

177

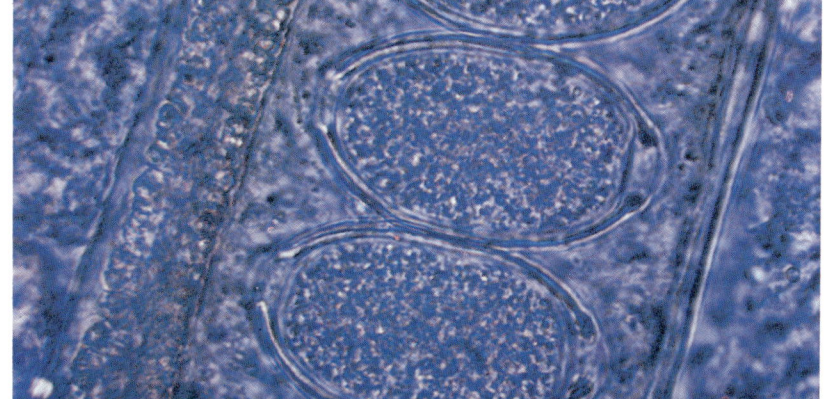

Coccidiosis

178 *Eimeria tenella*. Caeca of a young pullet distended with blood.

178

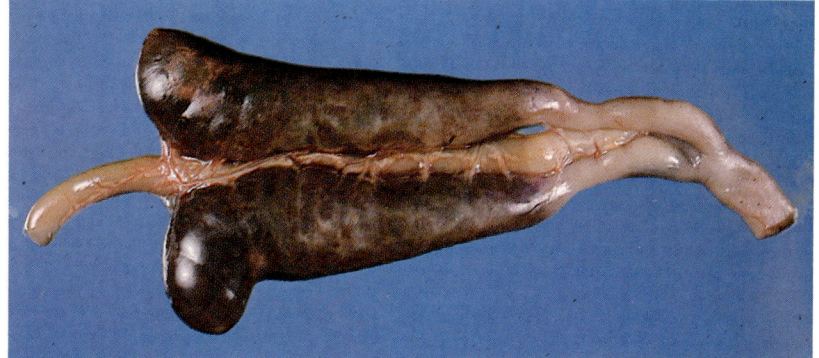

179 *E. tenella.* Extreme pallor of the pectoral muscles as a result of caecal haemorrhage.

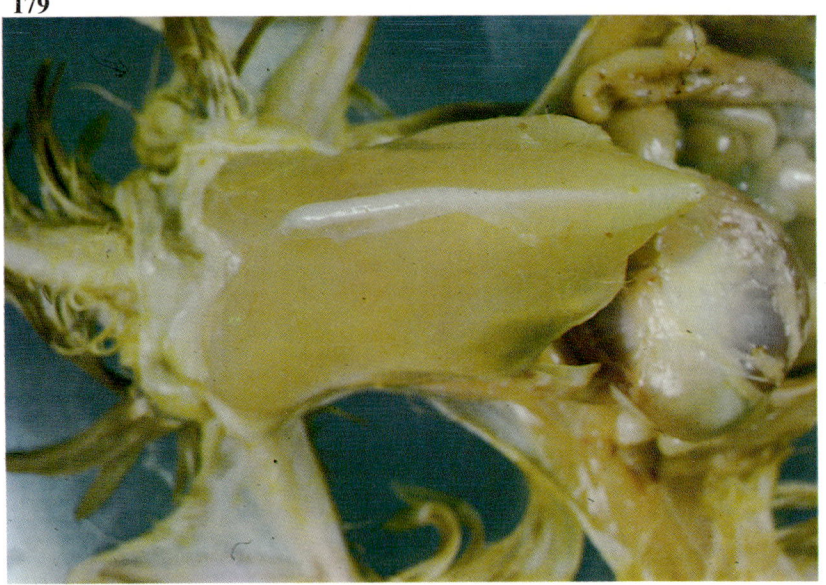

180 *E. tenella.* Caeca opened to show haemorrhagic debris. There may be firm caecal cores in subacute cases or in birds that are recovering. These cores are not usually adherent to the mucous membrane.

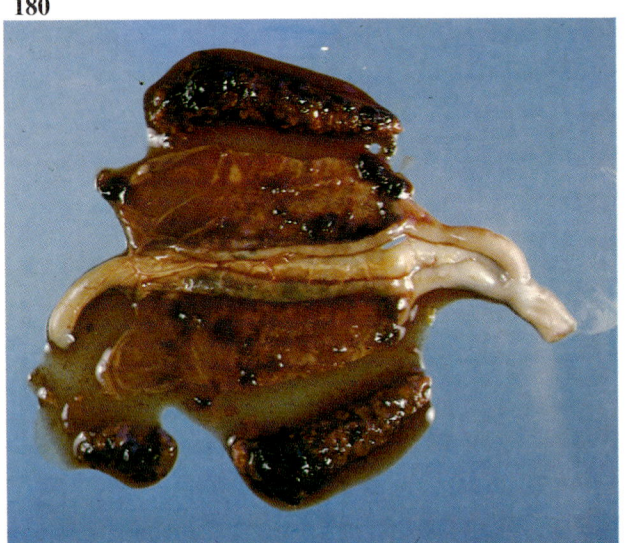

181 *E. tenella.* Smears of the haemorrhagic mucosa will demonstrate the large second stage schizonts. These are best viewed under a fairly low illumination of the microscope stage.

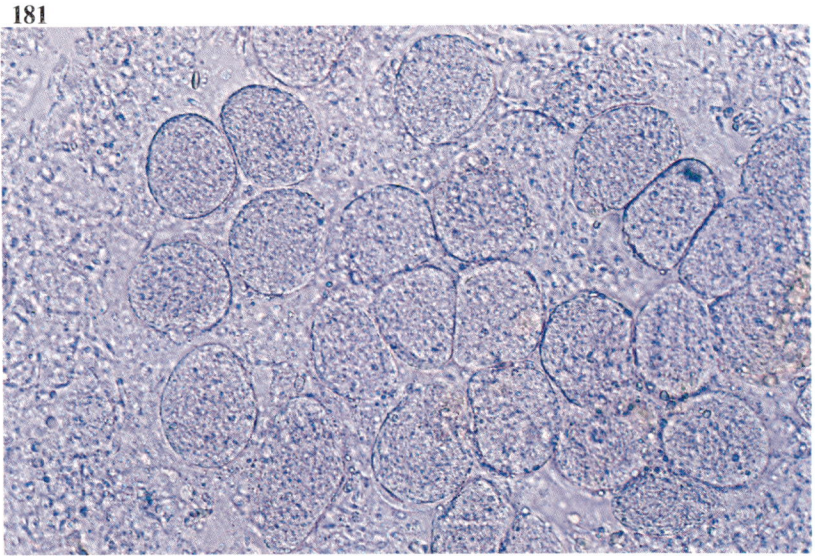

182 *E. tenella*. Second stage schizonts (containing merozoites) in disrupted caecal mucosa.

182

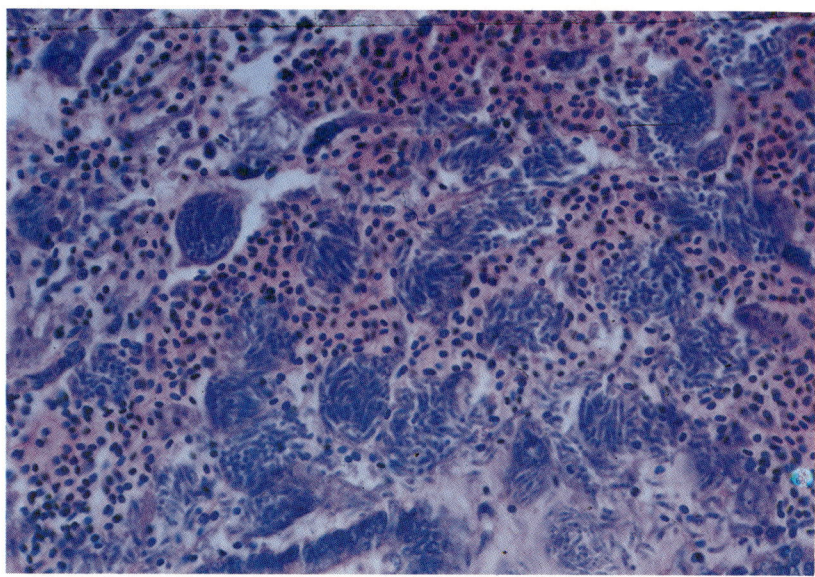

183 *Eimeria necatrix*. Distended small intestine showing mottled haemorrhages through the serous surface.

183

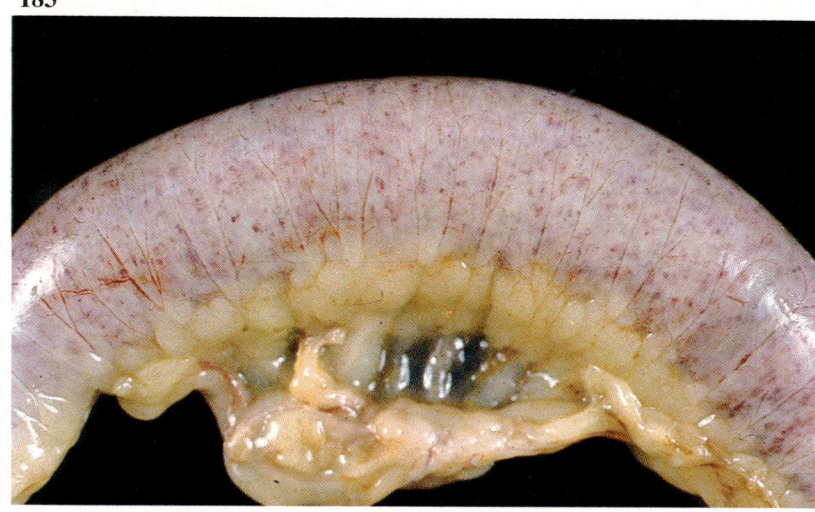

184 *E. necatrix*. Opened intestine from **183**. The lumen is full of mucoid debris. Haemorrhage is usually more pronounced. Mucosal smears show similar second stage schizonts to those observed in *E. tenella* infestations.

184

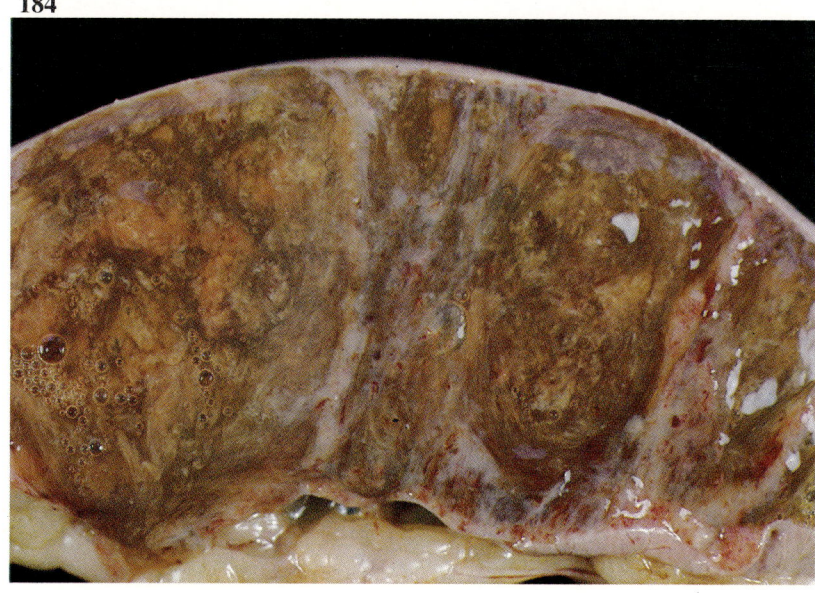

185 *E. necatrix*. Oocysts are found in the caecum and, in this photograph, are distending a crypt.

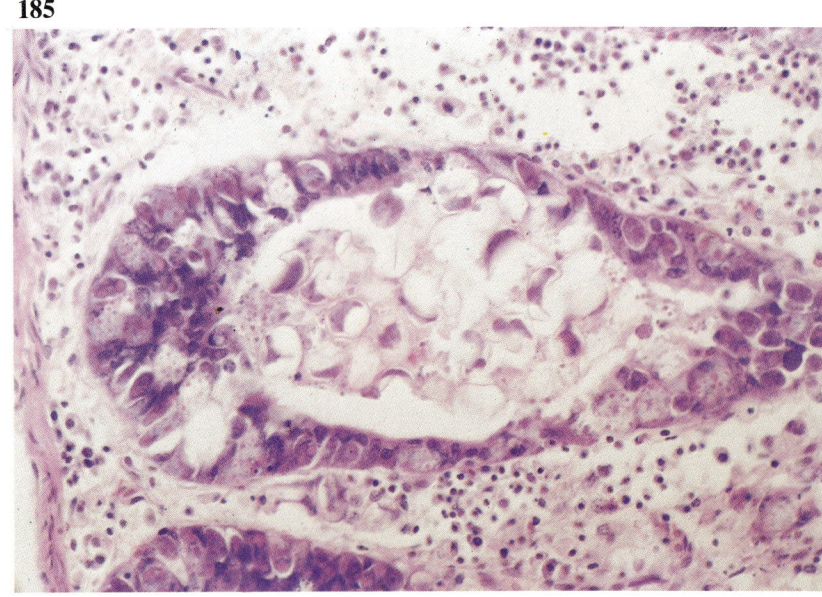

186 *Eimeria maxima*. Small intestinal mucus is often orangey-brown in colour.

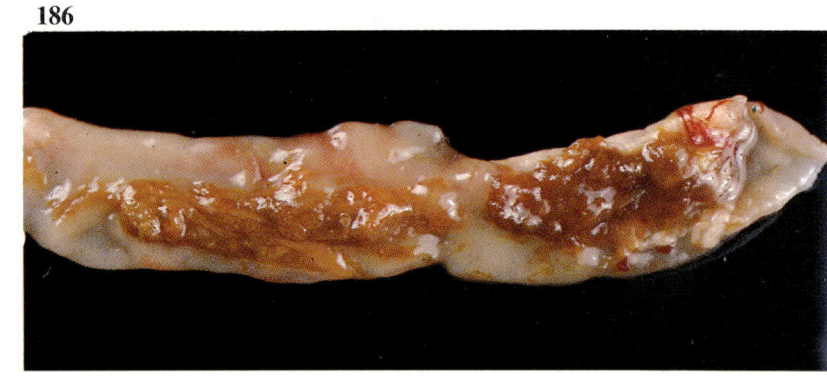

187 *Eimeria acervulina*. The mucosal surface of this intestine is roughened and slightly congested. The affected broiler breeder had concurrent lesions of Marek's disease. Small transverse white flecks can often be detected on the serous surface of the parasitised intestine.

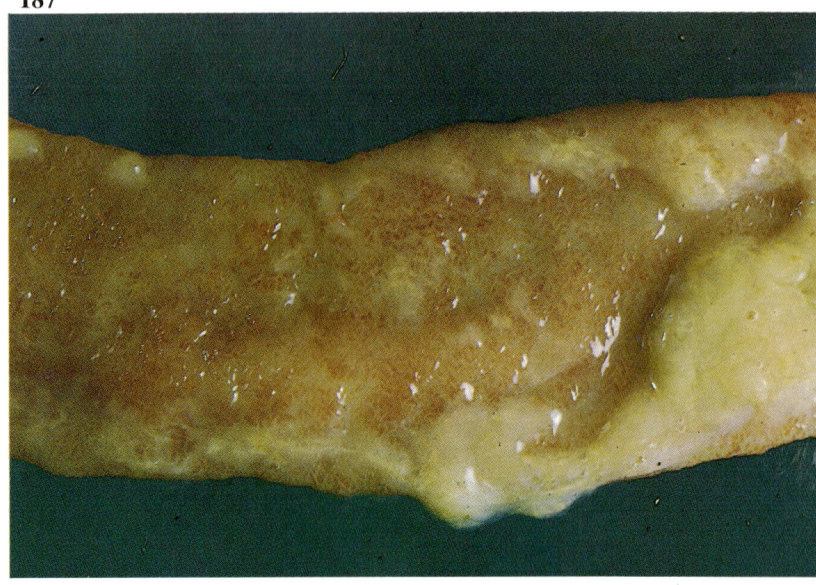

188 *E. acervulina*. Dense parasitisation of the small intestinal epithelium.

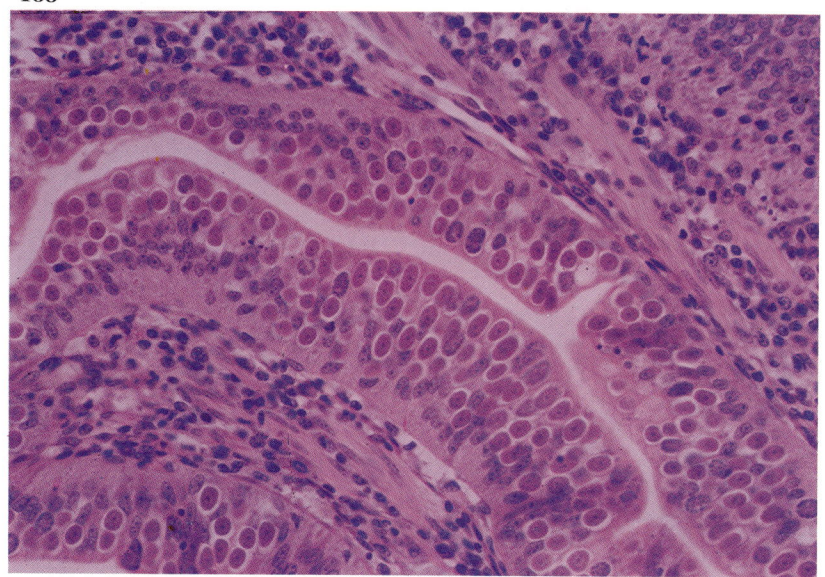

189 *Eimeria brunetti*. The lesions usually affect the lower part of the small intestine and the colo-rectum but can be more evenly distributed throughout the small intestine. This species causes severe necrosis of the superficial mucosa, which is difficult to distinguish grossly from uncomplicated cases of necrotic enteritis (*see* **37**). Secondary bacterial hepatitis may occur in birds that survive for more than a few days.

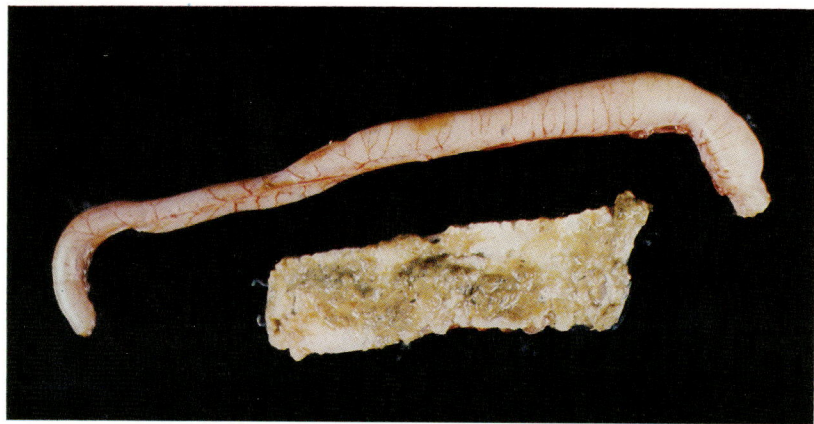

190 *Eimeria meleagrimitis*. The small intestine of this turkey poult is distended with pale fluid contents.

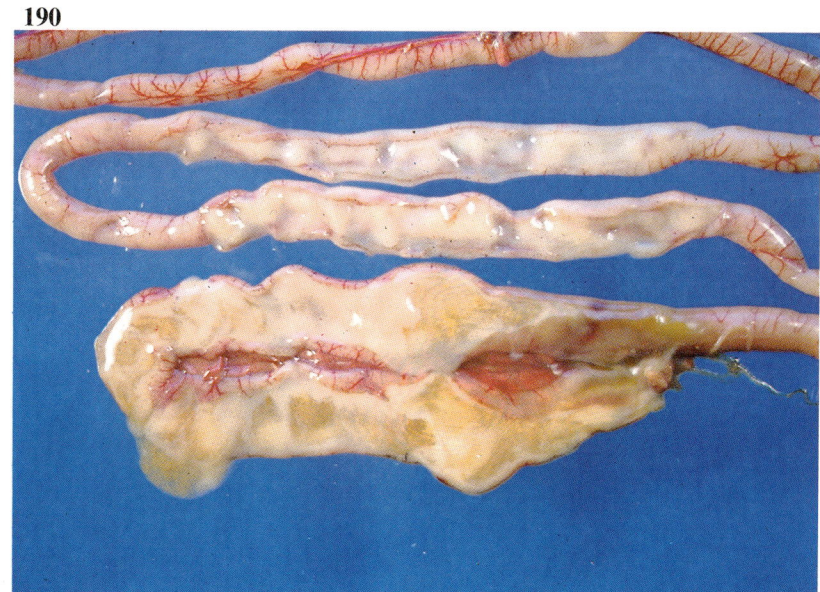

Histomoniasis *(Histomonas meleagridis)*

191 The disease is now a rarity in turkeys except in small flocks that have access to ground used by chickens. The caeca are distended with cores of inflammatory debris that are firmly adherent to the mucous surface. Localised peritonitis is often present. The focal liver lesions are rounded and have pale rings surrounding a darker central area. The condition occurs occasionally in the fowl.

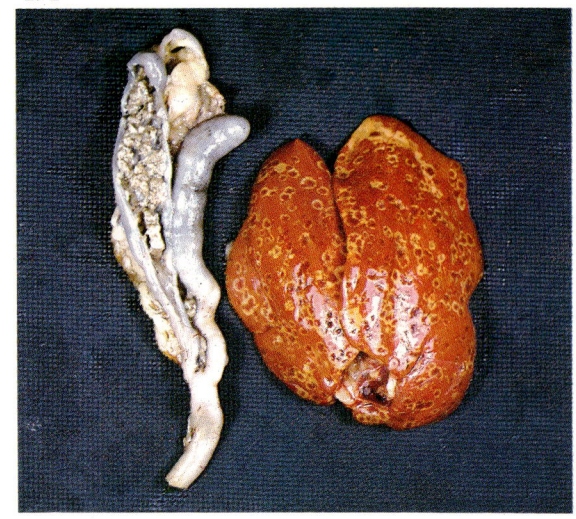

192 A section of an infected caecum shows the small rounded forms of the parasite. The histomonads may be more difficult to identify histologically in resolving lesions in the liver but should be readily seen during the acute stages. PAS-haematoxylin.

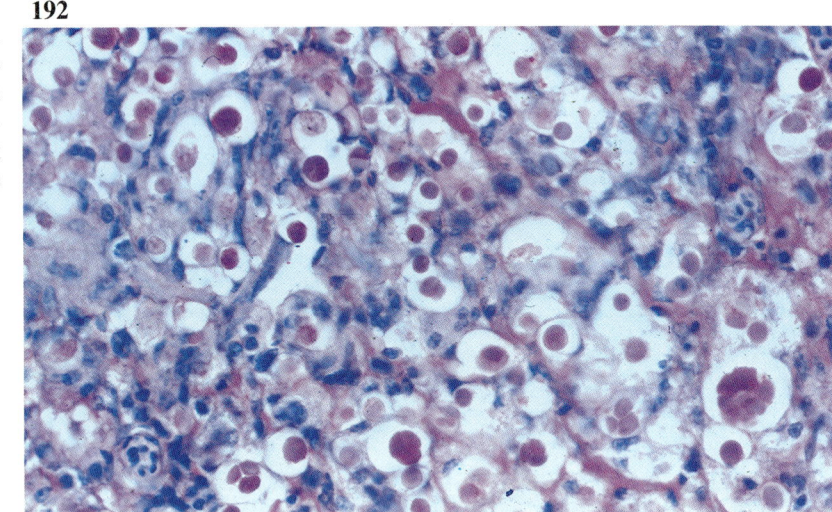

Cryptosporidiosis

193 The small basophilically staining parasites are present on the surface of the luminal epithelium in the bursa of Fabricius in a broiler. The epithelium is hyperplastic. Similar lesions may be observed in the trachea. No clinical signs were shown in this case but respiratory disease has been reported both in turkeys and in broilers. The small size of these organisms makes them difficult to see. They stain strongly with PAS.

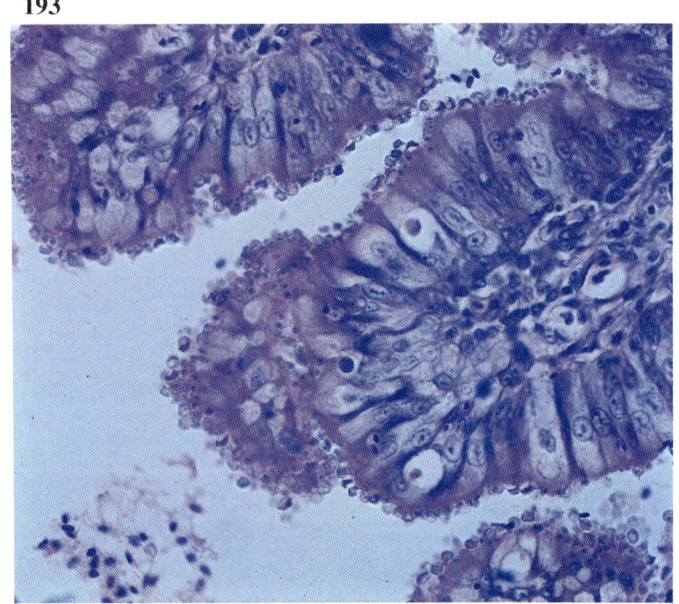

Scaly leg

194 The presence of the parasite *Knemidocoptes mutans* has caused the leg scales of a bantam to become raised due to the accumulation of debris underneath.

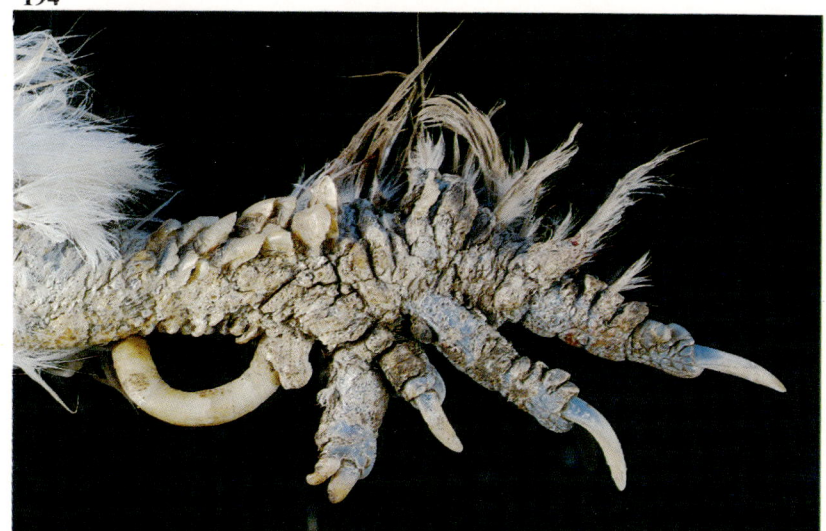

Lice

195 Large numbers of eggs (species unidentified) on feathers of a laying fowl from a flock where egg production was poor.

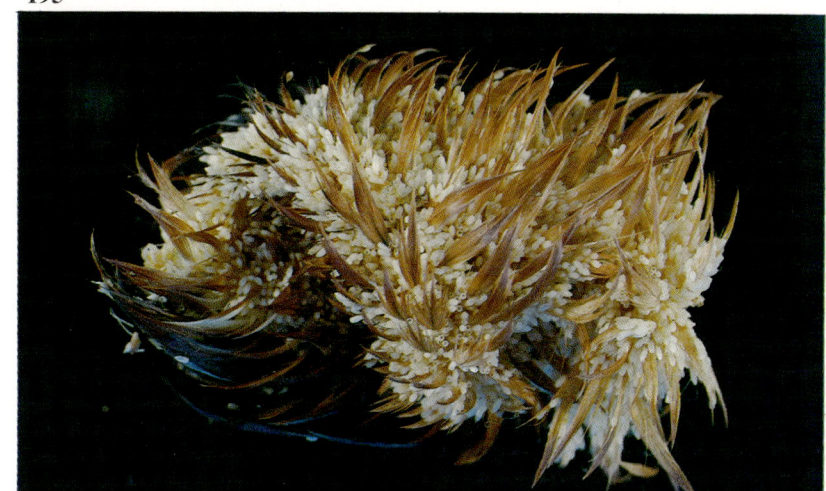

Red mite *(Dermanyssus gallinae)*

196 These parasites feed mainly at night and are usually found off the host. Their presence should be suspected in layers if egg production falls and anaemic birds are submitted for examination. Note the red colour of those mites that have recently fed. The mites are shown at about ten times life size.

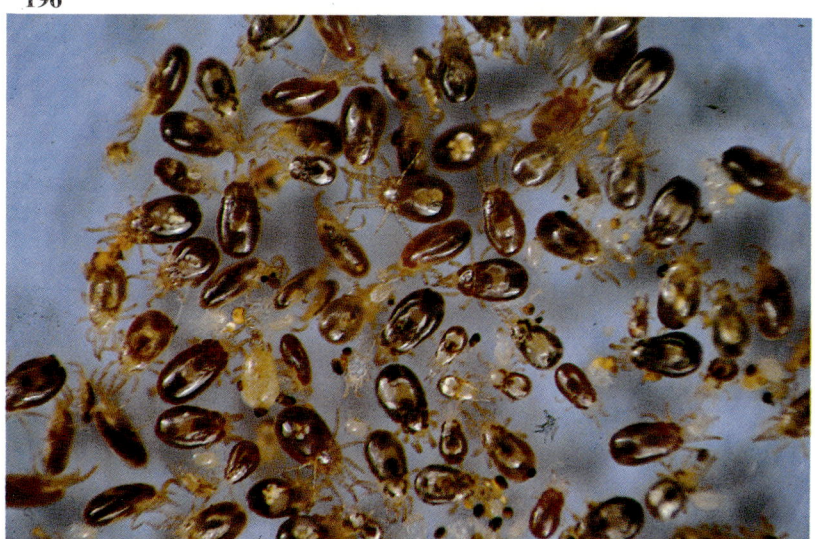

Northern fowl mite *(Ornithonyssus sylviarum)*

197 These mites live continuously upon the birds. They are seen here on the feathers of a broiler breeder that was submitted with excoriated tail and vent skin. These mites move quickly and are easily transferred to the gloves and arms of the person doing the post-mortem examination.

197

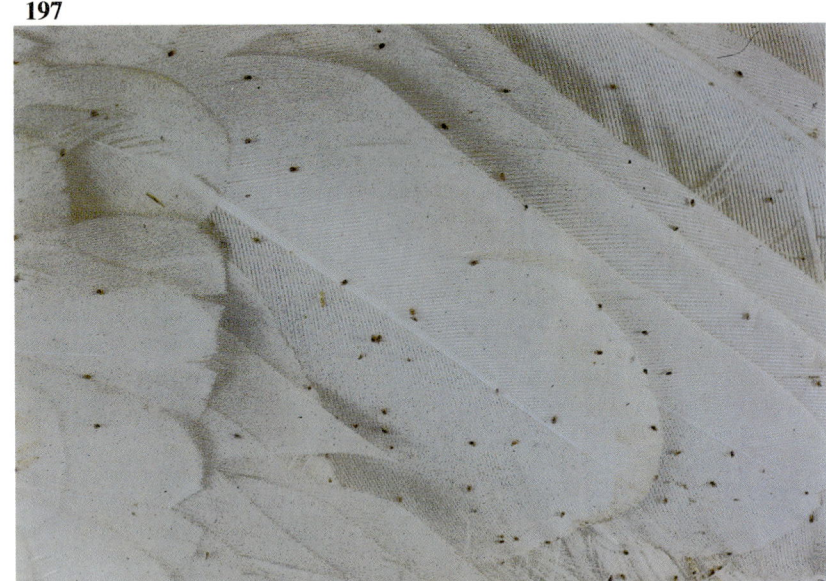

Nutritional deficiencies and metabolic disorders

Riboflavin deficiency

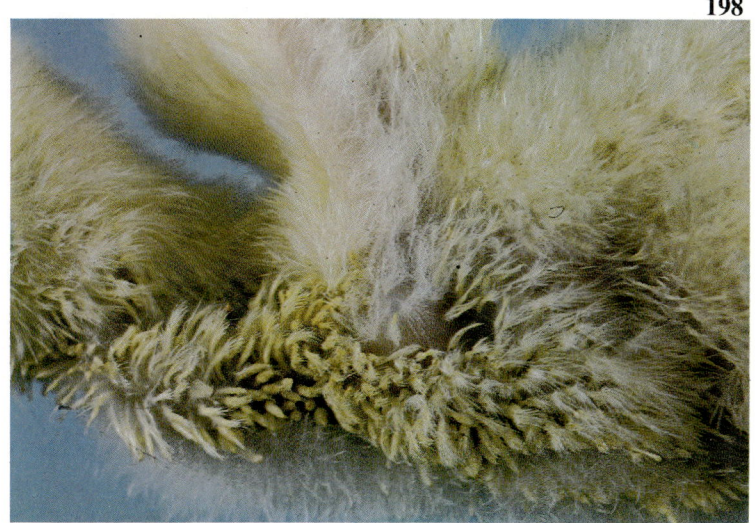

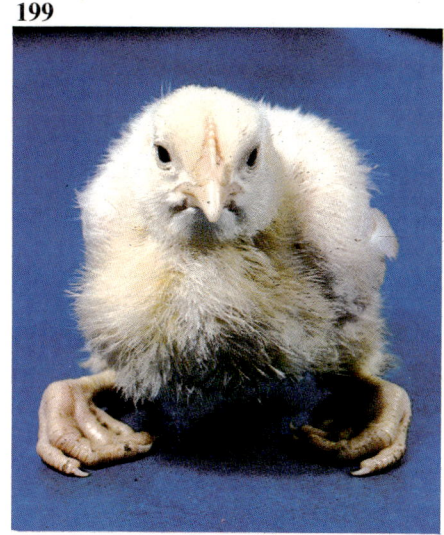

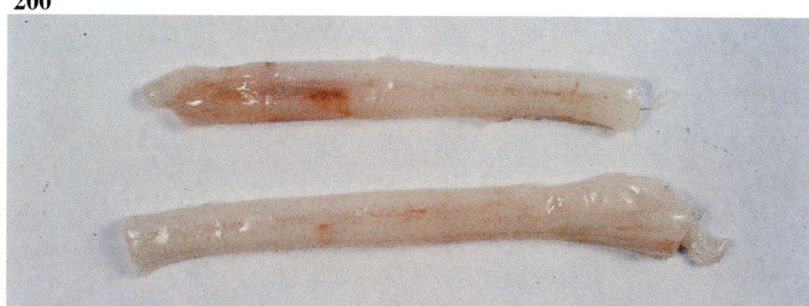

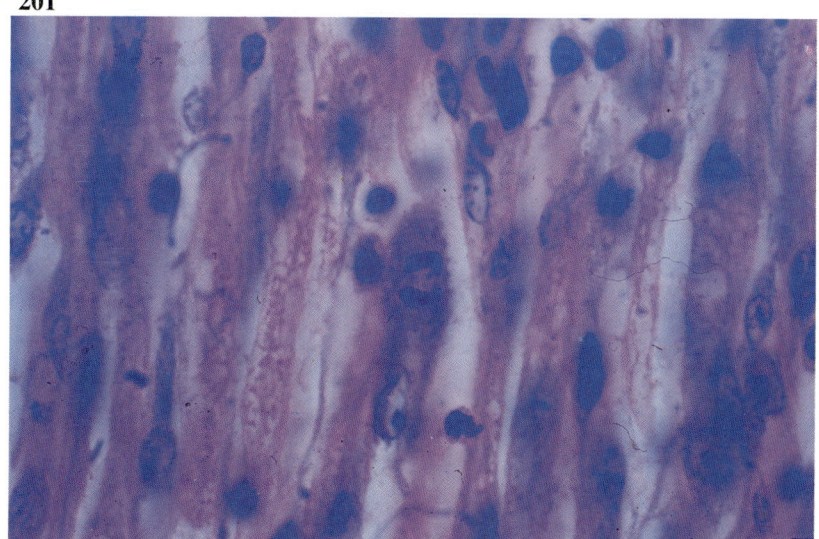

198 Clubbed down may occur in the unhatched embryos and day old chicks from parent flocks that receive inadequate levels of this vitamin.

199 Curled toe paralysis. Young chicks may show clinical signs at aproximately 10-14 days of age if they have been eating a deficient ration. The birds remain alert but are unable to rise from their hocks. They exhibit a flaccid paralysis and in-curling of the toes, which is not maintained after death.

200 The sciatic nerves are swollen and, on a white background, look discoloured.

201 Section of a sciatic nerve from a broiler chick with curled toe paralysis shows Schwann cell proliferation.

Encephalomalacia (crazy chick disease)

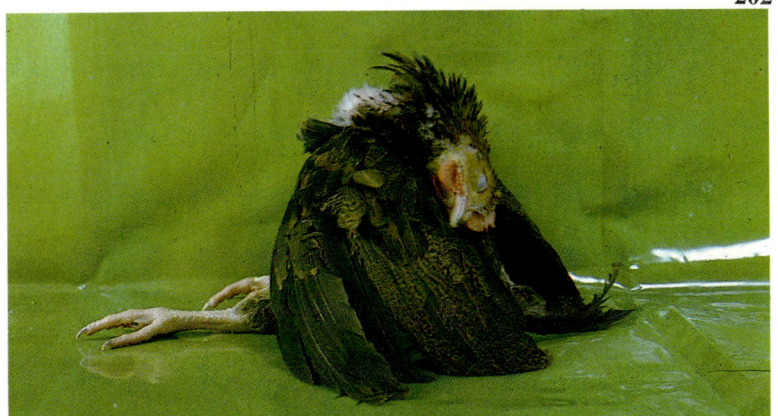

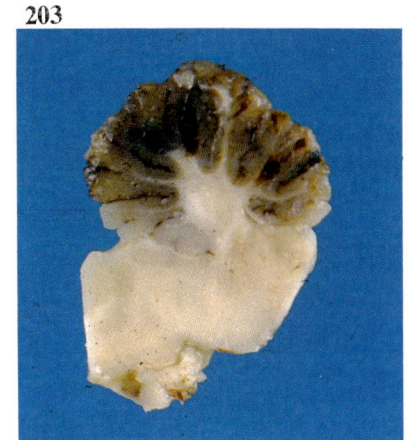

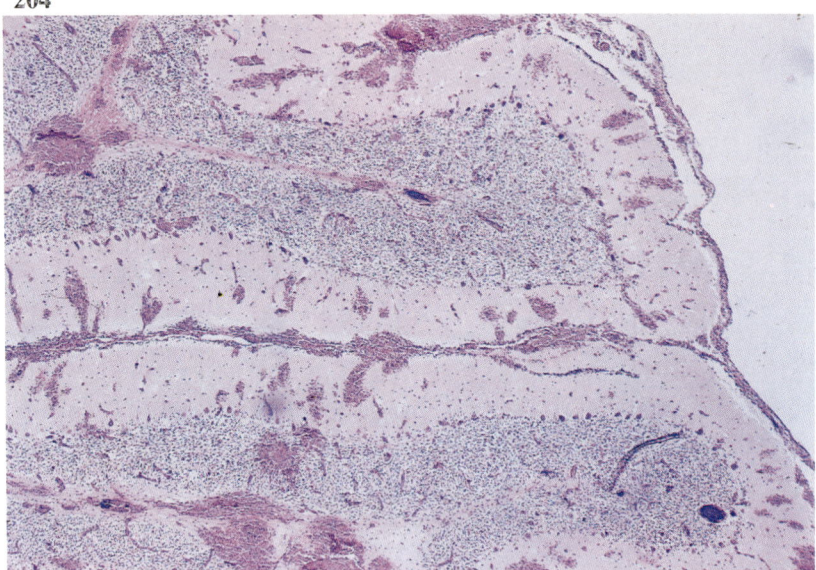

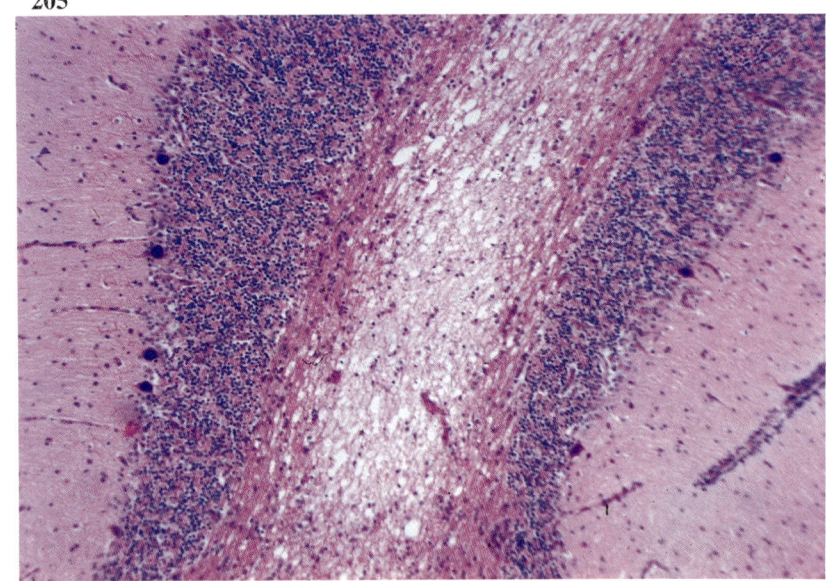

202 Opisthotonos in a 5-week-old pullet replacement. Clinical signs are most often seen between 2 and 3 weeks of age if chicks or turkey poults have been on a ration that is either deficient in vitamin E or one from which they are unable to obtain a sufficient amount of the vitamin.

203 Haemorrhage within a partly fixed cerebellum of a 2-week-old turkey poult. When present, gross lesions vary from extensive haemorrhage of the cerebellum to a barely detectable oedema and flattening of the cerebellar gyri and of the cerebral hemispheres.

204 Cerebellar haemorrhages. Haemorrhage usually occurs in severe lesions but it is not always present.

205 Focal malacic lesion in a cerebellar medullary ray. The malacia may be extensive or restricted to small punctate lesions, the latter being seen particularly in younger chicks. The lesions are most frequently observed in the cerebellum and brain stem but can also affect other parts of the brain.

206 Hyaline capillary thrombi are often associated with the malacic foci. Martius scarlet blue.

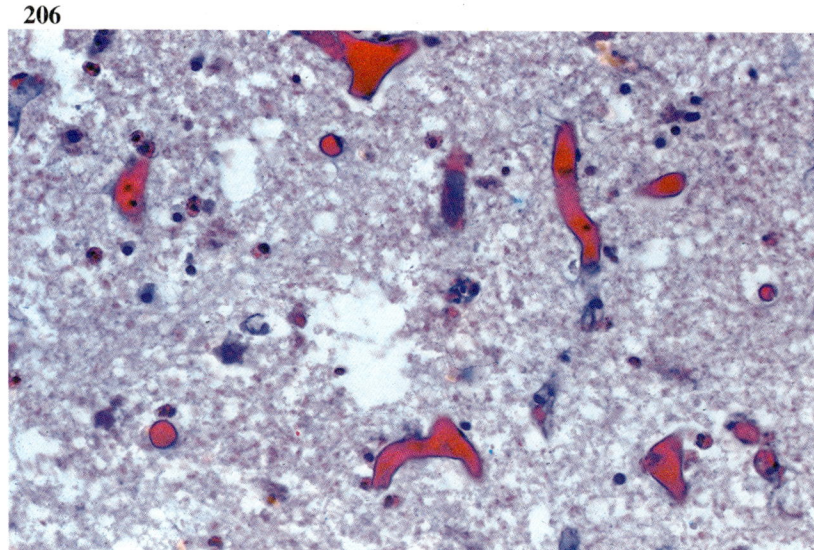

Rickets

207 Rickety rosary in a 3-week-old chick. Field outbreaks appear to occur more frequently in turkey poults. The condition is usually caused by a deficiency of vitamin D but may also be produced by a lack of calcium or phosphorus or by an imbalance of these two minerals. An inability to rise from the hocks and severe depression are the principal clinical signs.

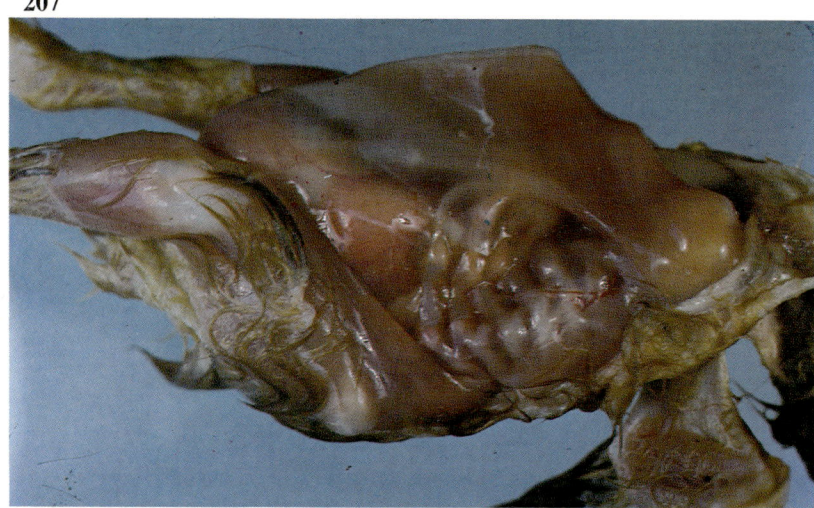

208 Beading of the rib heads is a common feature.

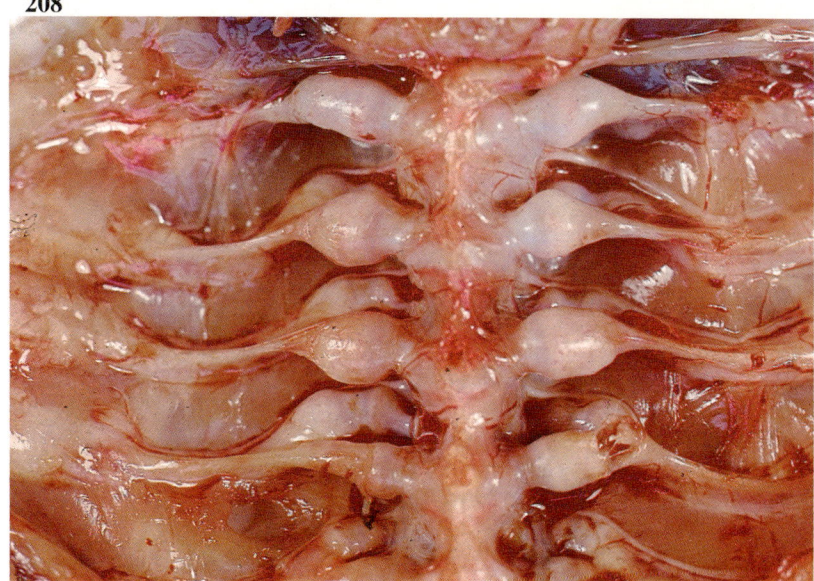

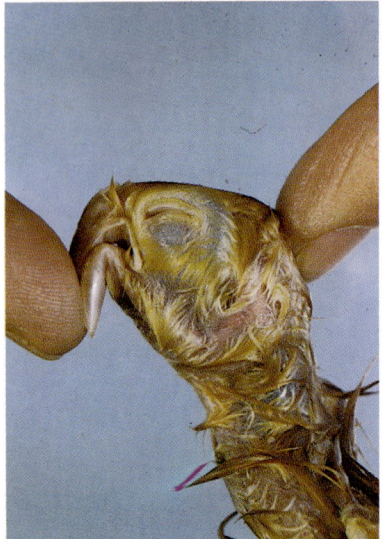

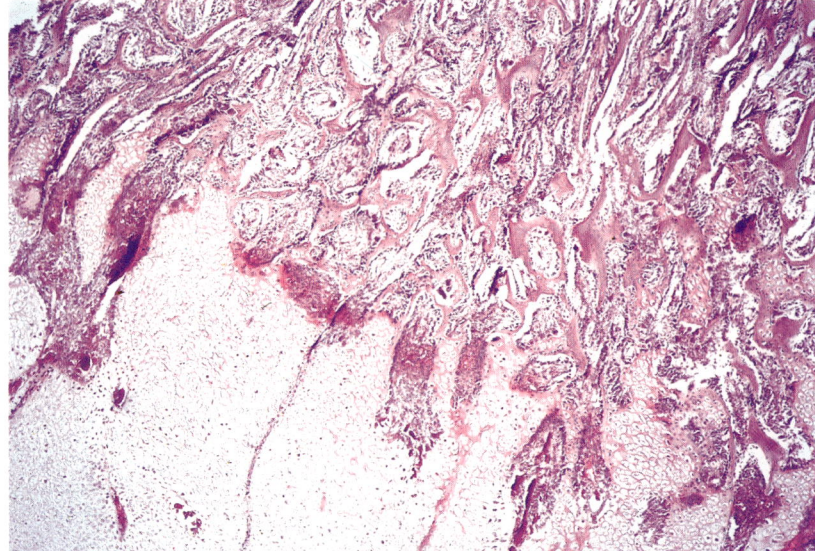

209 Post-mortem assessment of bone strength may be difficult in any bird under 2 weeks of age but in rickets the tarsometatarsi are usually rubbery and do not break cleanly under pressure. Displacing the beak also provides a good indication of the strength of the facial bones.

210 The growth plate cartilages of the long bones are often thickened and poorly penetrated by blood vessels.

211 The columns of cartilage cells in the growth plate may be irregularly aligned. 3-week-old pheasant PAS-Alcian blue.

212 The parathyroid glands are sometimes markedly enlarged. This section shows a cord-like arrangement of parenchymal cells and proliferation of stromal connective tissue from a severe case in a 3-week-old broiler. Acrylic resin, Lee's methylene blue-basic fuschin.

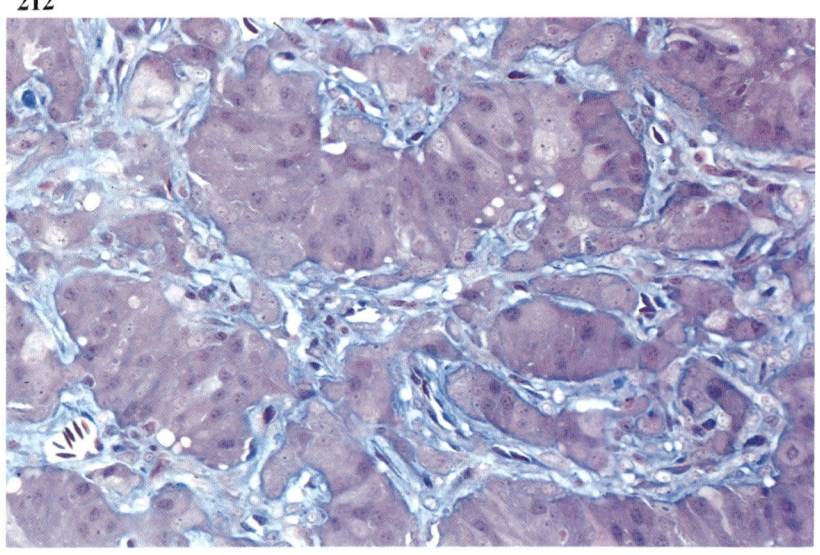

Calcium deficiency in adult laying fowl

213 Twisted sternum. The sternum and rib cage are frequently soft and distorted. Egg production drops and the shells are thin.

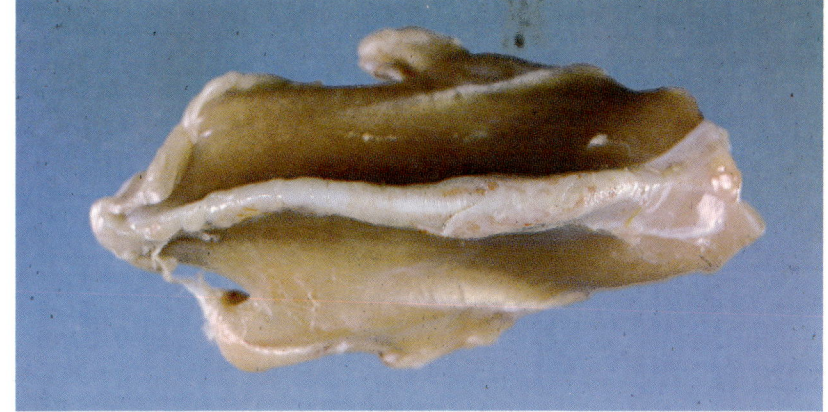

214 Sigmoid flexure of the ventral part (arrows) of two ribs caused by pathological fractures.

214

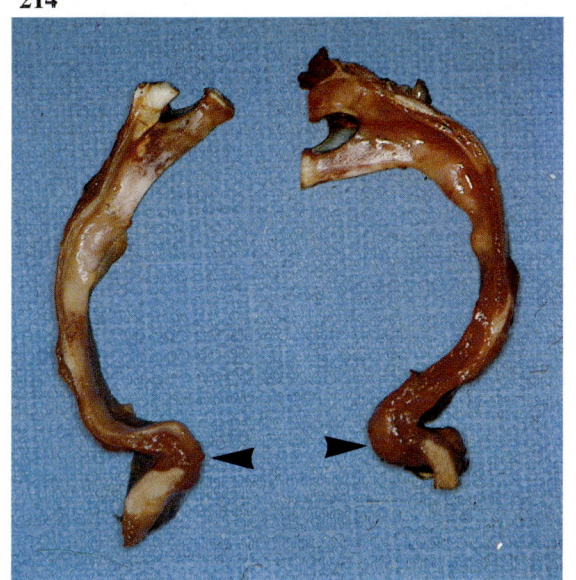

215 Fractured rib seen in **214**. One cortex is shown.

215

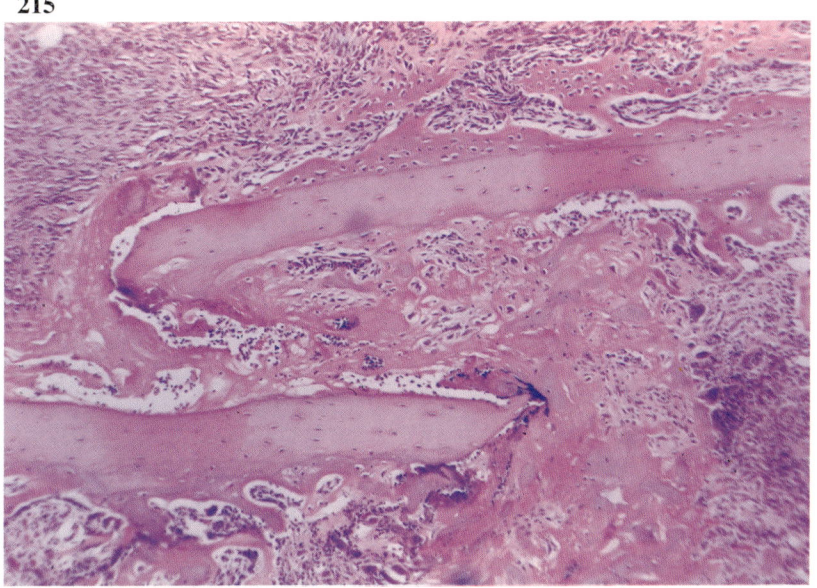

Fatty liver and kidney syndrome

216 The condition has been traditionally associated with broilers but has also been known to cause mortality in commercial layer chicks. Such chicks are seen here with ruffled feathers, depression and some are unable to rise from their hocks. Outbreaks of the condition have been largely prevented by the inclusion of additional biotin in rations.

217 The subcutaneous fat is congested. This feature gave rise to the name 'pink disease'.

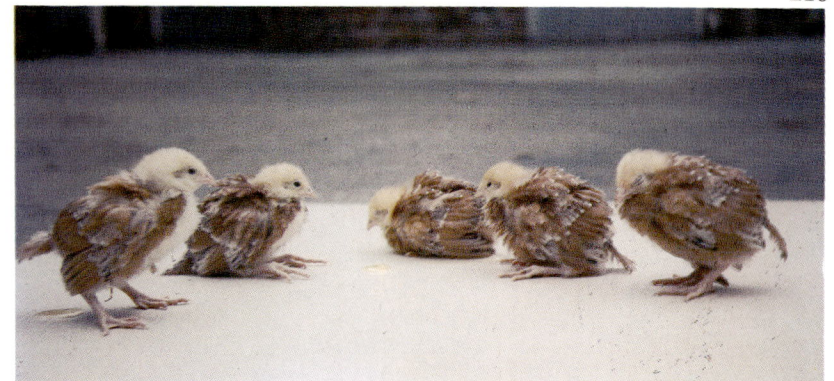

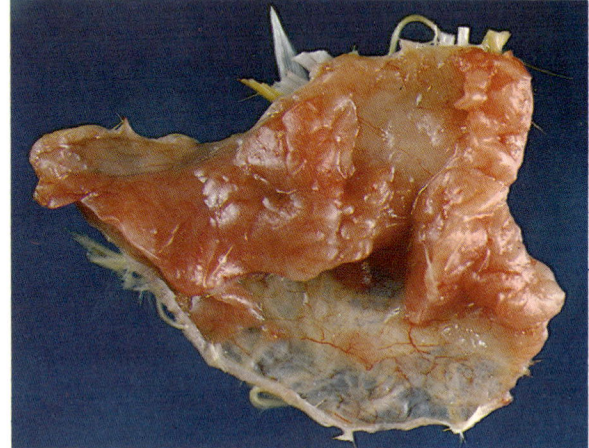

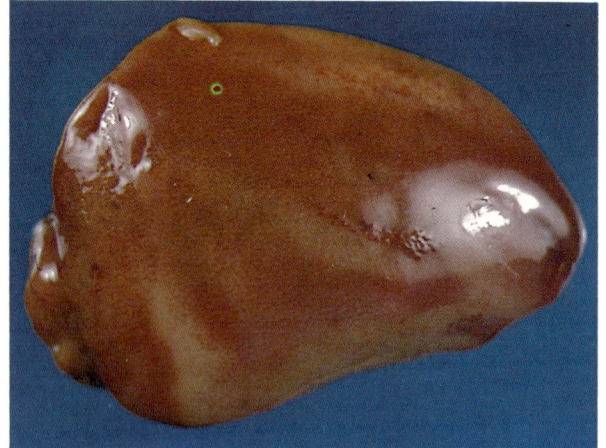

218 Livers are pale, often in a rather streaky fashion, and friable. It may be difficult to cut blocks of this tissue for fixation.

219 Subcapsular haemorrhages may be present at necropsy. Although it is not demonstrated in this specimen such haemorrhages are usually clustered near the posterior tips of the lobes (*see* **90**).

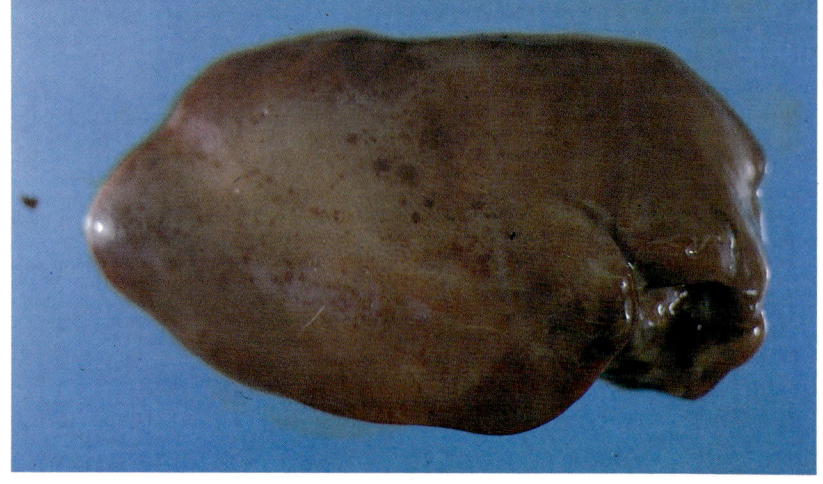

220 Most kidneys contain pale areas of tissue which contrast with the deep reddish brown colour of the normal organ. The kidney of this broiler was severely affected and had an even pallor. Note the outline of individual lobules within the renal divisions.

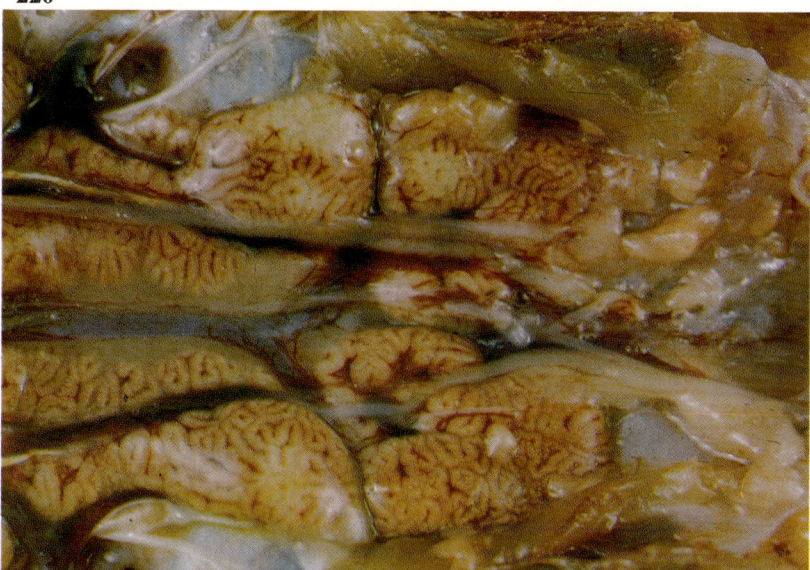

221 A pale heart (left) from an affected broiler contrasts with the normal colour of the organ in an older bird.

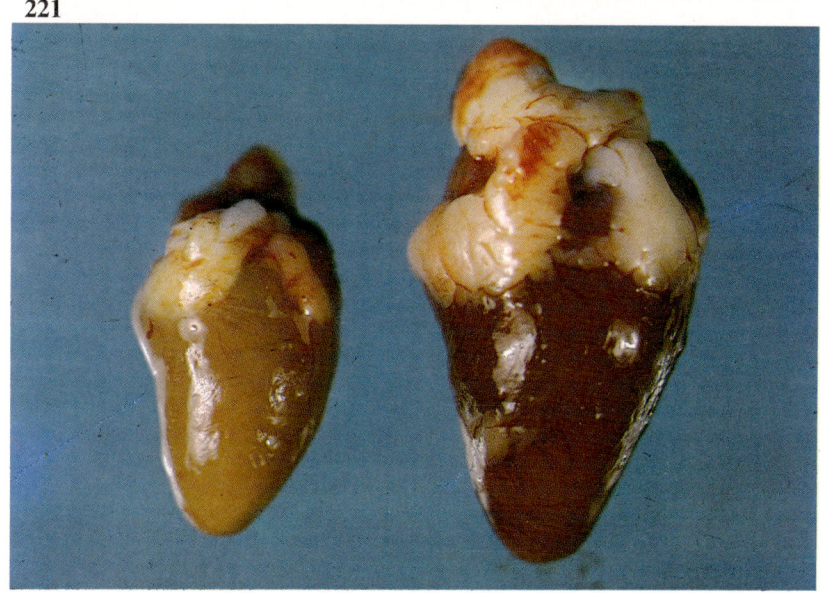

222 The small intestinal contents, especially those of the duodenum, may be very dark and possess a strong odour.

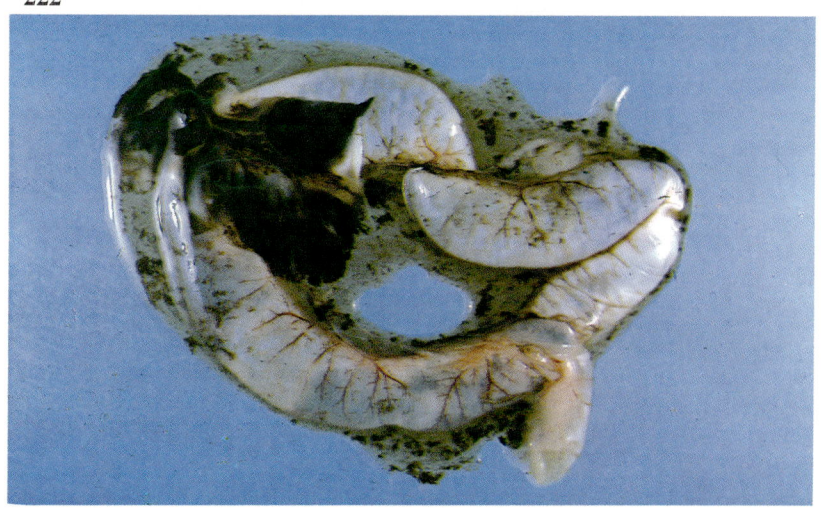

223 A large quantity of fine lipid droplets are contained within the proximal convoluted tubular cells of this kidney. Oil red O. Histological confirmation of this disease requires demonstration of lipid in the kidney, liver and heart.

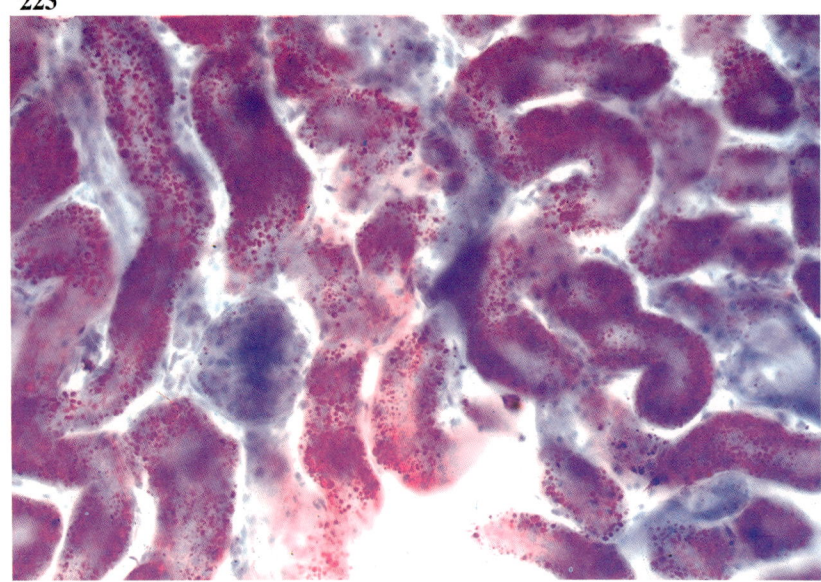

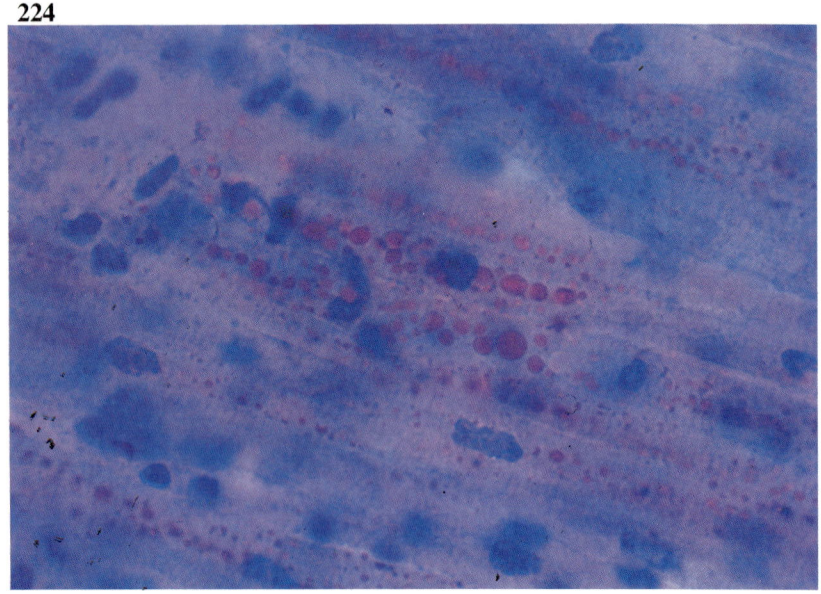

224 Fat droplets within the myocardium of a broiler. Oil red O.

Diseases of uncertain or unknown aetiology

Fatty liver haemorrhagic syndrome in laying fowl

225 A large blood clot surrounds the ruptured right lobe of the liver in a obese layer. Note haemorrhages in the unruptured left lobe. The bird may survive several haemorrhagic episodes, particularly if escaping blood is confined within the lobes or as a subcapsular haematoma. The condition occurs in obese birds; both metabolic and environmental associations have been implicated.

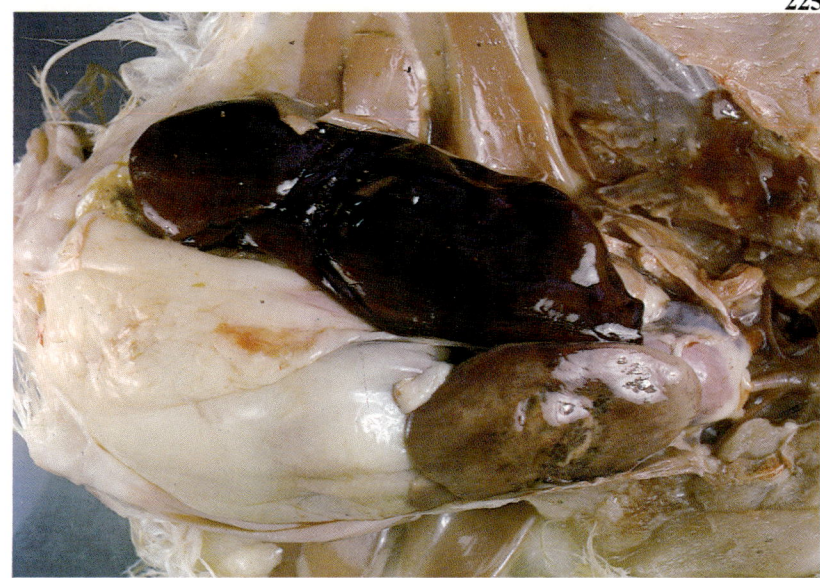
225

226 A large abdominal blood clot arising from the ruptured liver of an adult commercial layer. Note the pale comb in the decapitated head of the same bird.

226
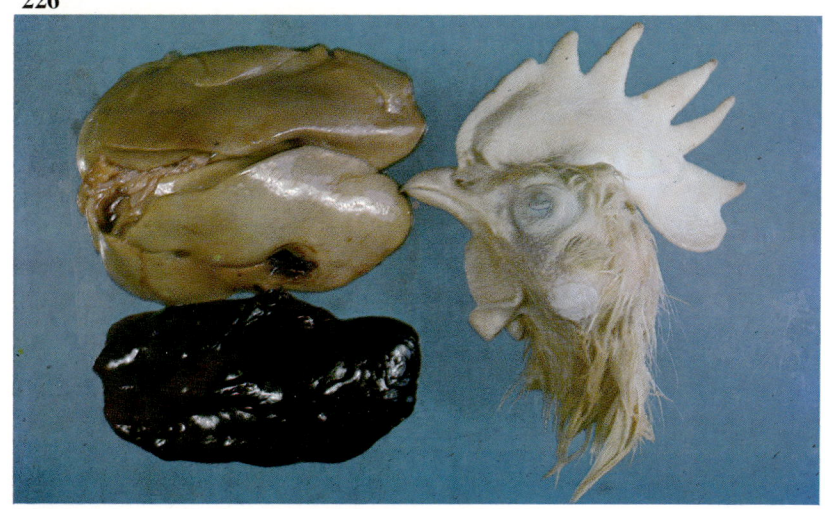

227 Cut surface of one liver lobe. The block was taken in an area where haemorrhage had not occurred. The tissue is usually extremely friable and it can be difficult to obtain suitable blocks for histology. It is usually better to put large portions into fixative and trim after 24 hours.

227
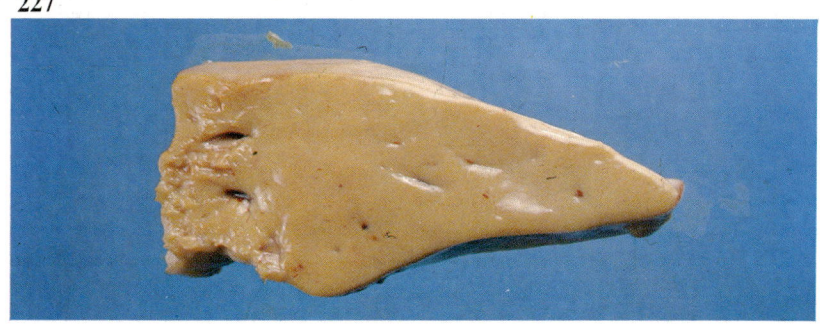

228 Excess fat in the ruptured liver of an obese layer. Sudan IV.

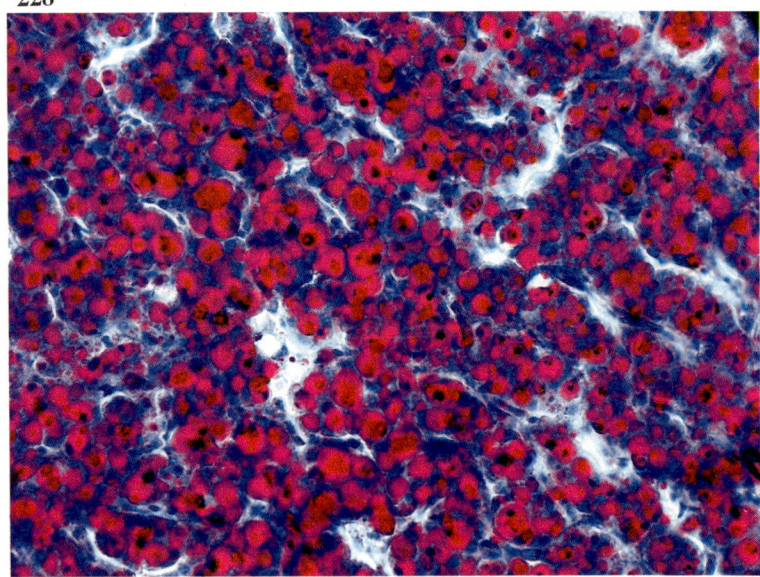

229 Death may occur in obese layers without haemorrhage taking place. Fine droplets of lipid are exuding through the liver capsule. Note the pad of abdominal fat.

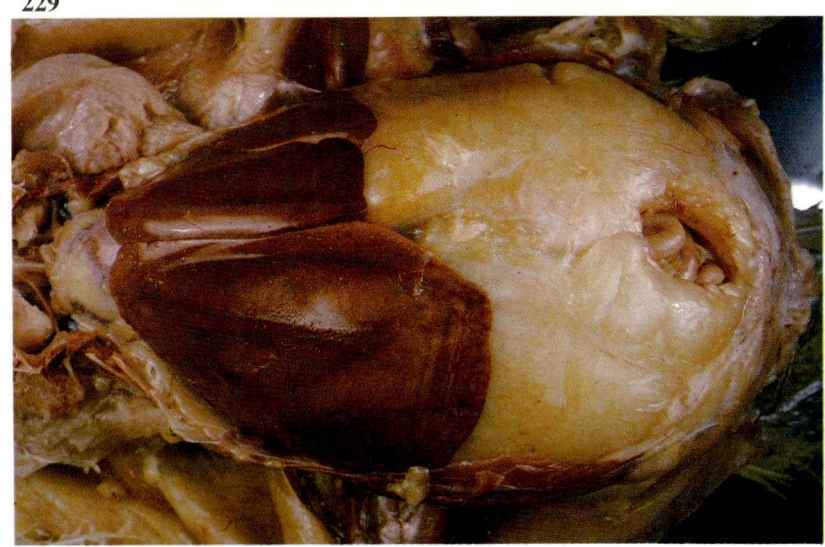

230 The presence of reticulin is demonstrated in the blood vessel walls but not in the surrounding parenchyma. The lesion has been described as a reticulolysis. Gordon and Sweet.

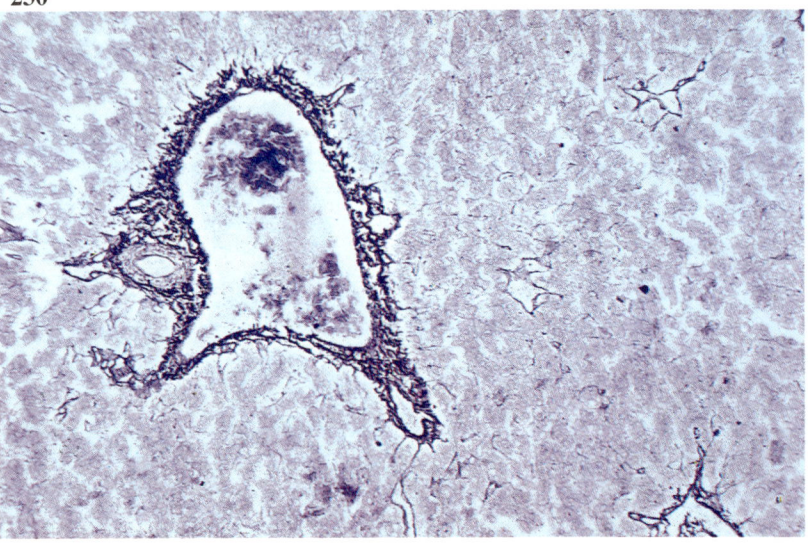

231 Reticulin network in normal liver demonstrated by the same technique as in **230**.

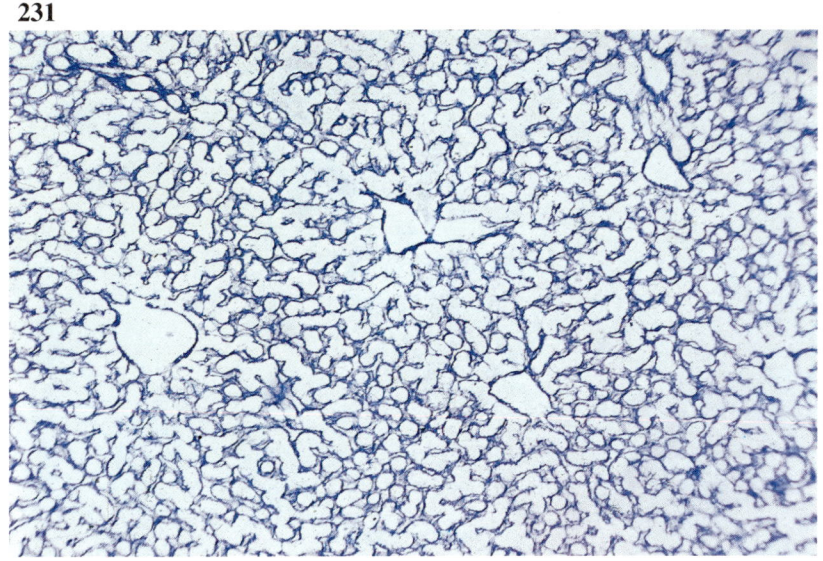

Sudden death syndrome in broilers ('acute heart failure', 'flip-over')

232 This syndrome may cause death in broiler flocks from the end of the first week onwards. Males are more frequently affected than females. Most carcases are found on their backs. Note the good condition of this carcase and the lack of any muscular congestion.

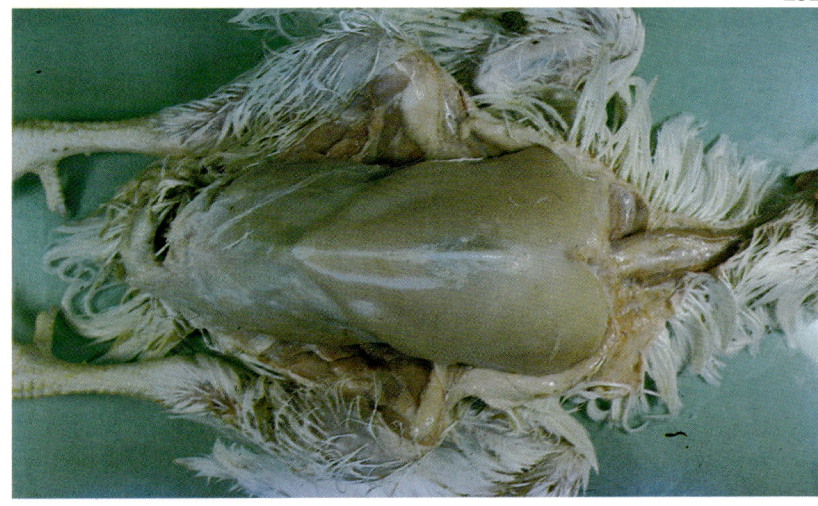

233 Bilateral pulmonary congestion and oedema is the principal finding at necropsy. The digestive tract is full of food and there may be some pallor of the intestine, liver and kidneys.

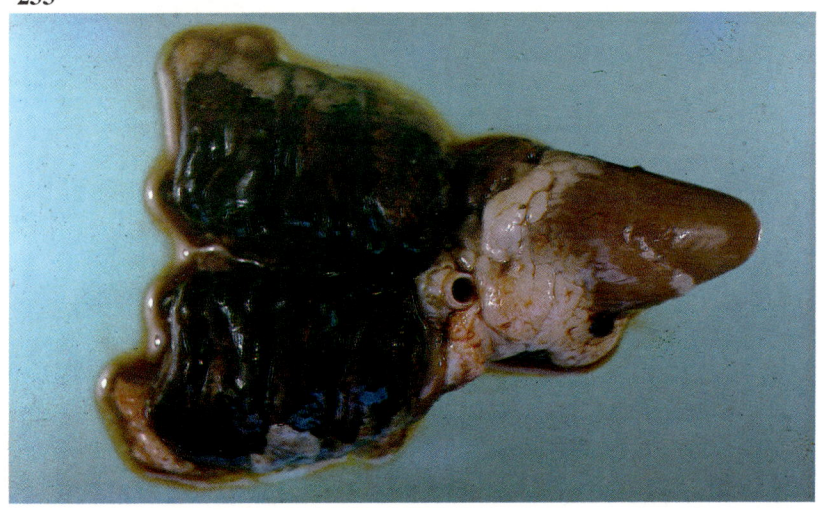

234 Pools of serosanguinous fluid often remain between the ribs after the lungs have been removed.

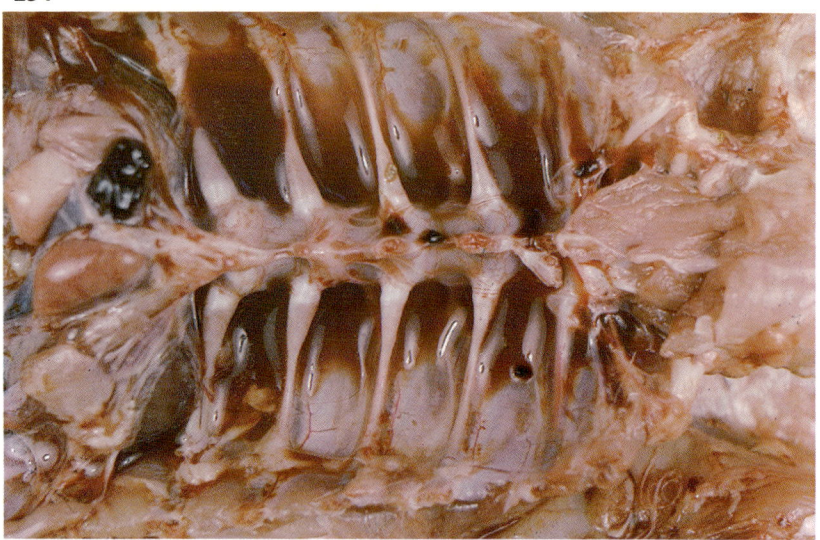

235 A section of lung confirms the intense congestion seen *post mortem*. The airways are full of proteinaceous fluid (arrows). There may be haemorrhages in the mucosa of the secondary bronchi.

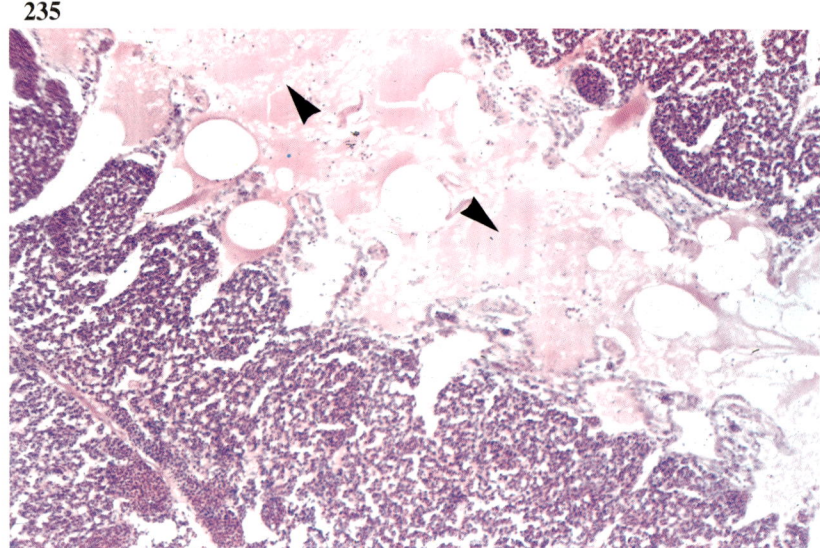

Sudden death syndrome in laying fowl

236 A common cause of sporadic death in both commercial and breeding birds that are in full lay. Protrusion of congested cloacal tissue through the vent is the only external feature.

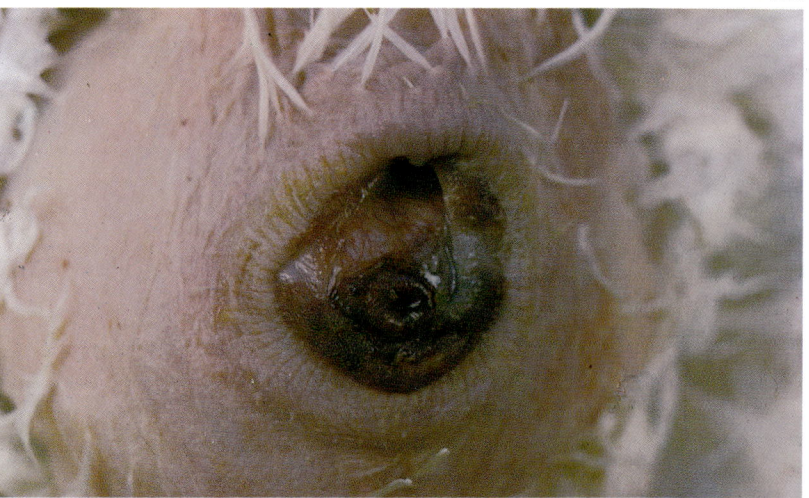

237 Intense congestion of the blood vessels on the surface of the ova and variable pulmonary congestion are frequently seen as post-mortem features. A broken, shelled egg is sometimes found in the shell gland.

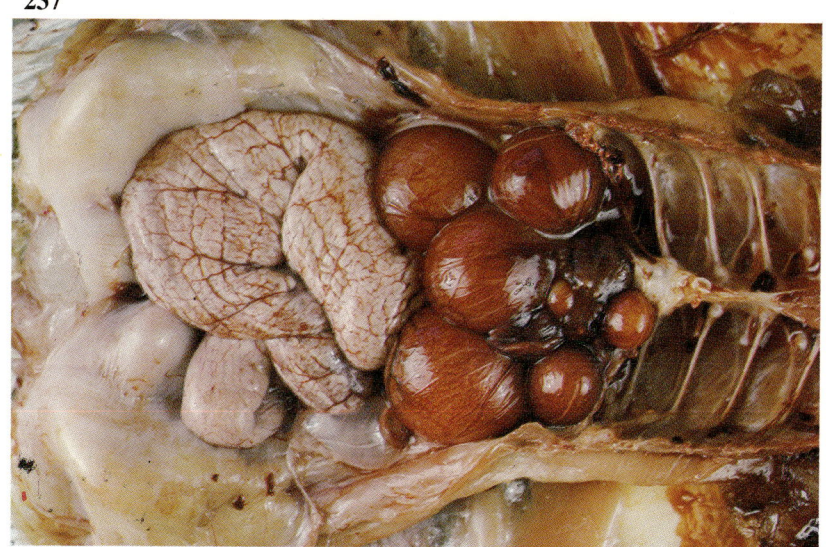

Cardiohepatic syndrome in turkey poults ('hepatosis')

238 Typically, the syndrome occurs at 7-10 days of age but may be seen up to 3 weeks of age. Poults are not usually seen ill and are found dead. Dilation of the right side of the heart, ascites, a pale slightly 'brittle' liver and generalised venous congestion are the main post-mortem features. The relationship of this condition to the appearance of similar gross lesions in older turkeys is uncertain.

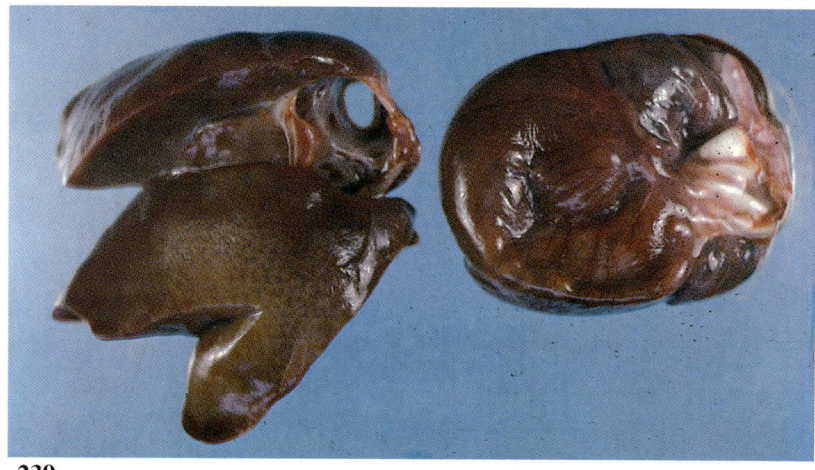

239 Liver sections reveal non-fatty vacuolation of hepatocytes and the presence of round PAS-positive cytoplasmic bodies. PAS-haematoxylin.

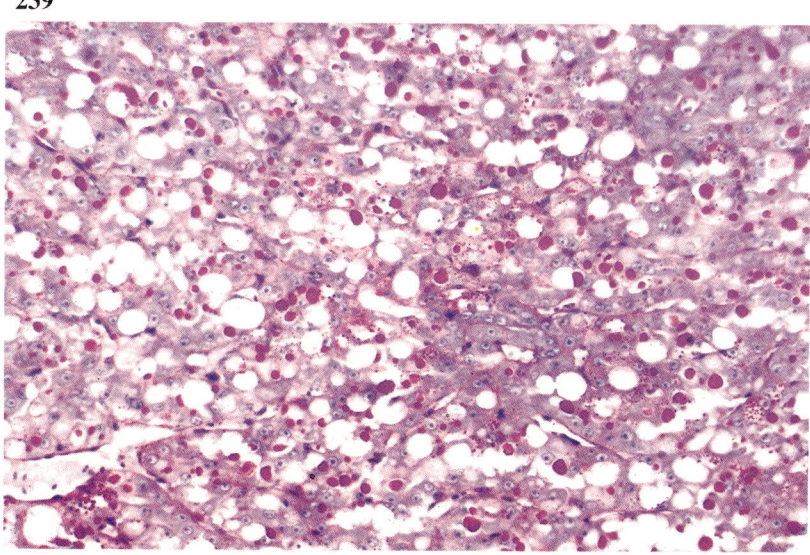

240 The rounded cytoplasmic bodies within degenerating hepatocytes also stain eosinophilically. One such body (arrow) is seen near the centre of this photograph.

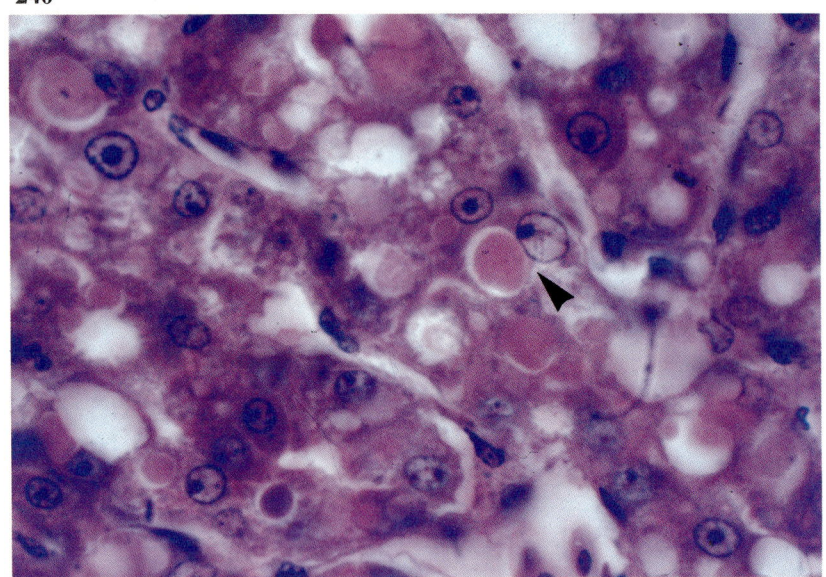

Ascites and congestive heart failure in broilers

241 A common condition mainly occurring in male broilers. Frequently seen as an incidental finding in many flocks but there may be occasional outbreaks. There is severe ascites and a marked passive venous congestion throughout the carcase. Note the deep red colour of the musculature.

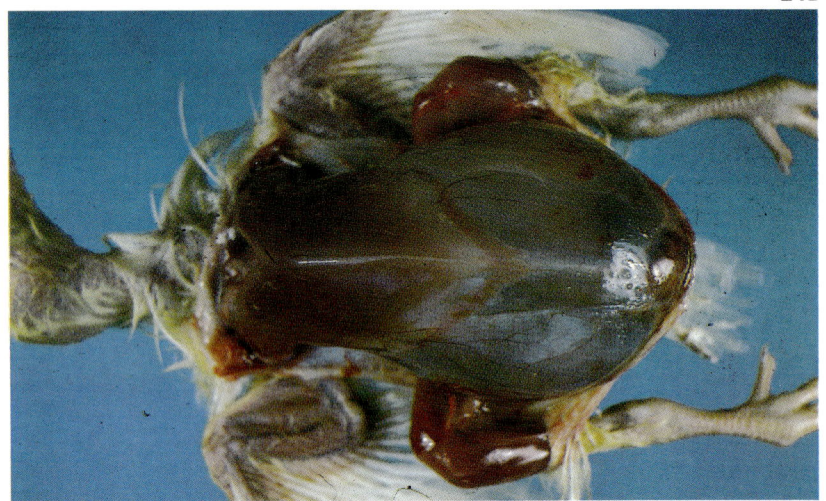

242 The ascitic fluid may be semi-clotted. The liver is small and has rounded borders. Dilation of the right side of the heart and intense passive congestion of the lungs and other viscera are the main findings. The terminal stages are analogous to congestive heart failure.

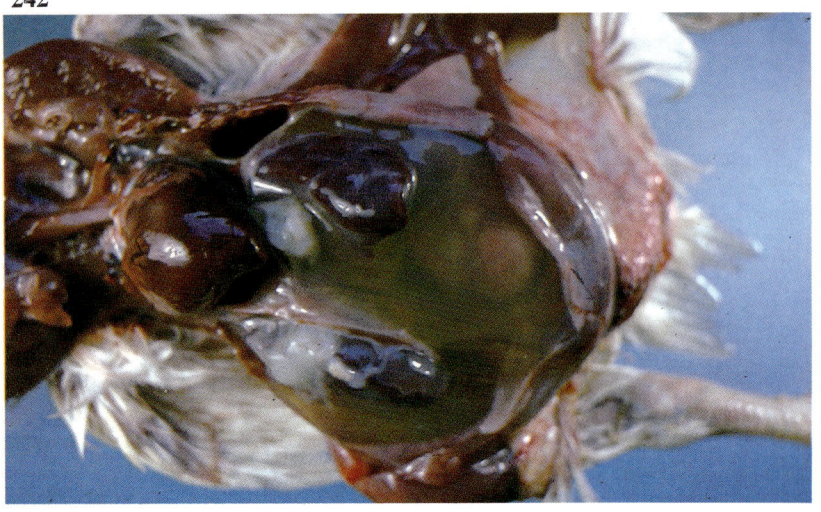

243 Comparison of an affected liver (left) with a normal organ.

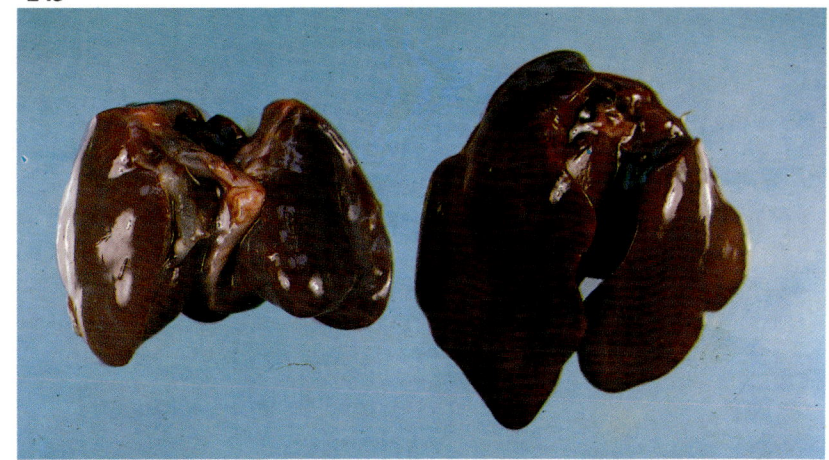

244 Low power view of a chronic liver lesion. A fibrinous deposit on the surface of the liver is partly organised. Other features not seen in this photograph include dilation of the intrahepatic branches of the hepatic vein and a variable increase in parenchymal connective tissue. Martius scarlet blue.

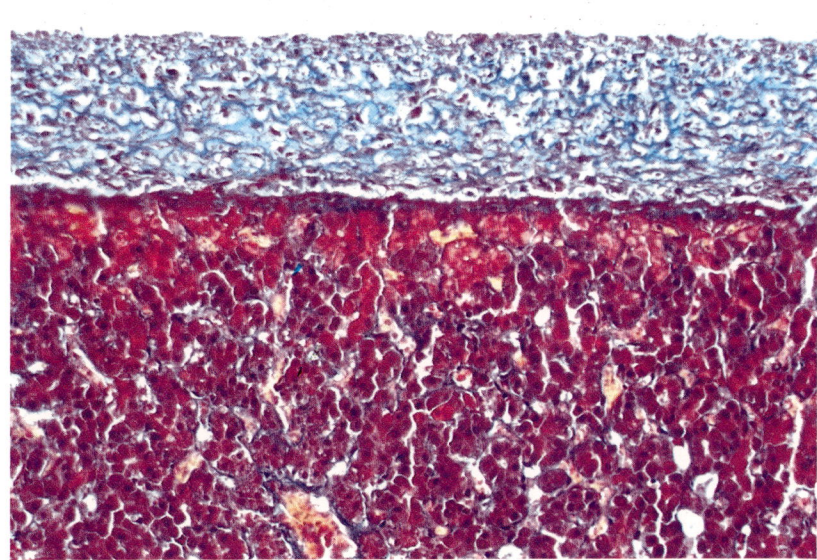

245 Dead birds are also found in affected flocks with hepatic lesions that may represent an earlier stage of the condition. Grossly, such livers are swollen, discoloured and often have a mottled or dimpled surface. In this specimen dimpling is not present but a fine reticular pattern of pale bands of tissue can be seen through the capsule.

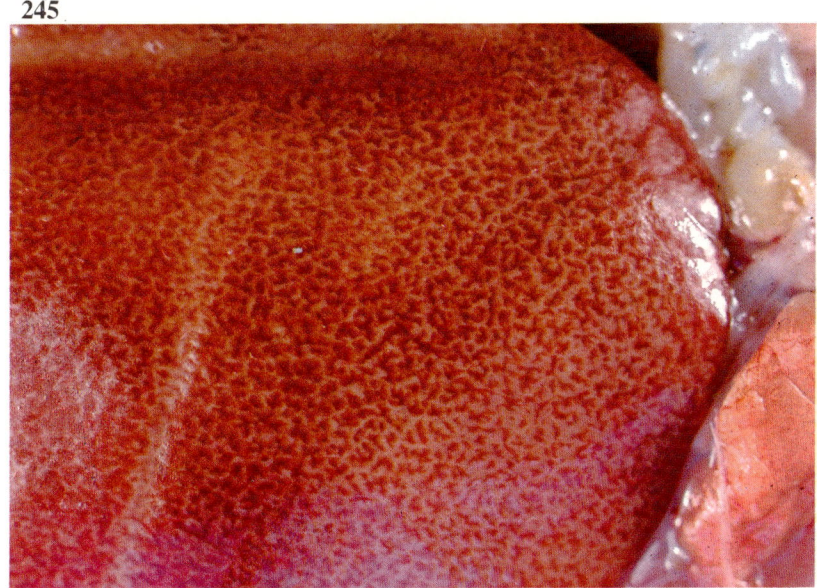

246 Sections from a liver such as that in **245** reveal, initially, a marked hepatocytic fatty change that mainly affects periacinar tissue. This is quickly succeeded by coagulative necrosis of the affected zones. Here, a central band of surviving hepatocytes is flanked by degenerating cells on either side, vacuolation (fatty) is apparent at the junctions (arrows) of the viable and degenerating hepatocytes. Haemorrhagic replacement and heterophilic infiltration are variable features of such lesions.

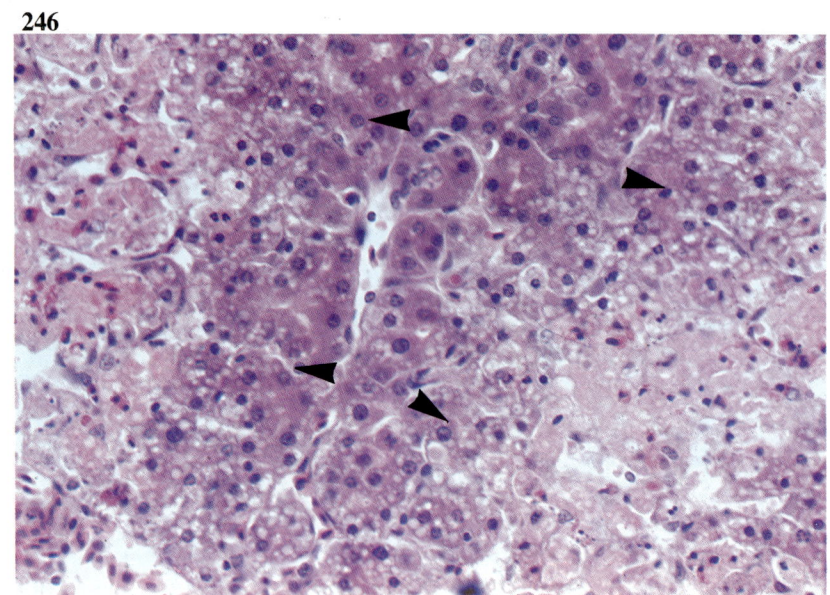

Round heart disease

247 This condition is now uncommon but at one time was seen as a cause of sudden death during winter months in fowls maintained on deep litter. The enlarged heart usually has a blunted apex in which there may be a central depression.

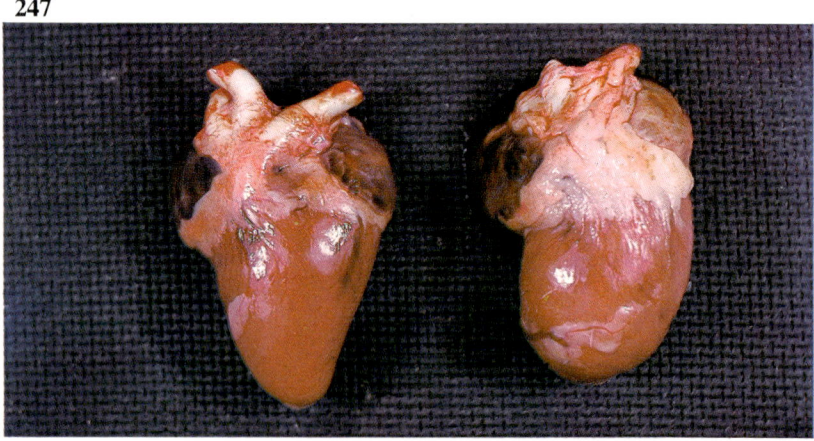

248 Degenerative fatty changes in swollen heart muscle fibres cut in cross section. Note also nuclear degeneration.

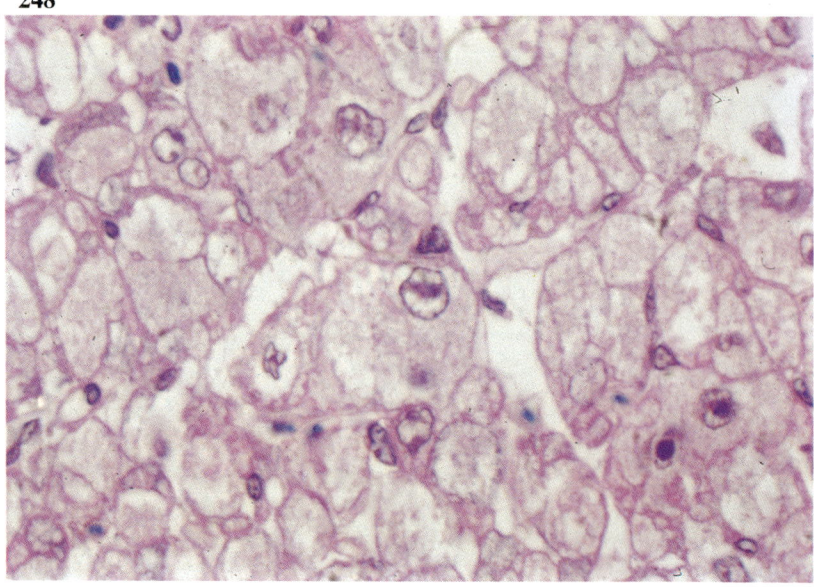

Dyschondroplasia

249 Seen in both broilers and turkey growers. It is more common in male birds. This cartilage abnormality may be present at the ends of all the long bones in the leg and has been reported in the humerus. The tibiotarsus is most frequently affected and in this 6-week-old broiler the upper part of the bone is severely deformed.

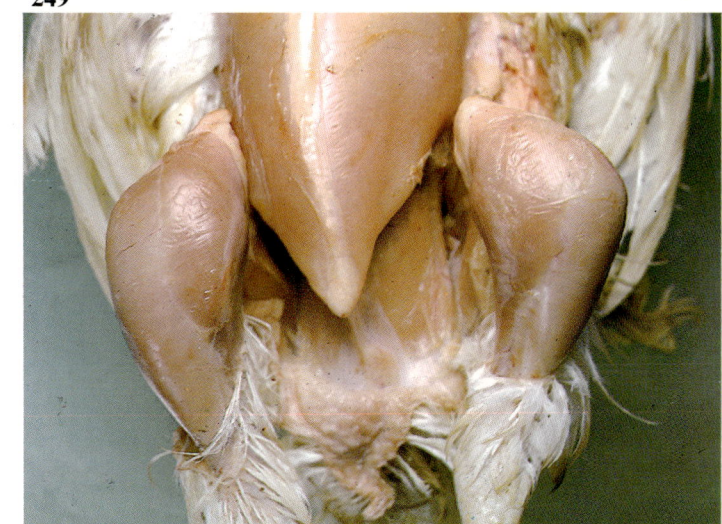

250 The top bone is a tibiotarsus removed from the broiler in **249**. It has been split to show the large posteriorly bent head containing a plug of abnormal cartilage (arrows). Pathological fractures are present on both the anterior and posterior aspects. The bone below is normal.

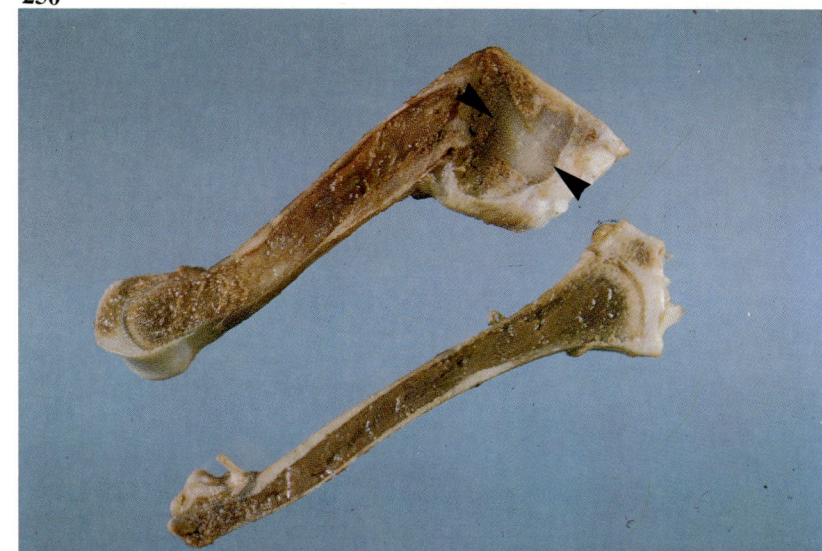

251 The head of this tibiotarsus is also bent posteriorly. A large mass of abnormal cartilage extends from the growth plate into the metaphysis.

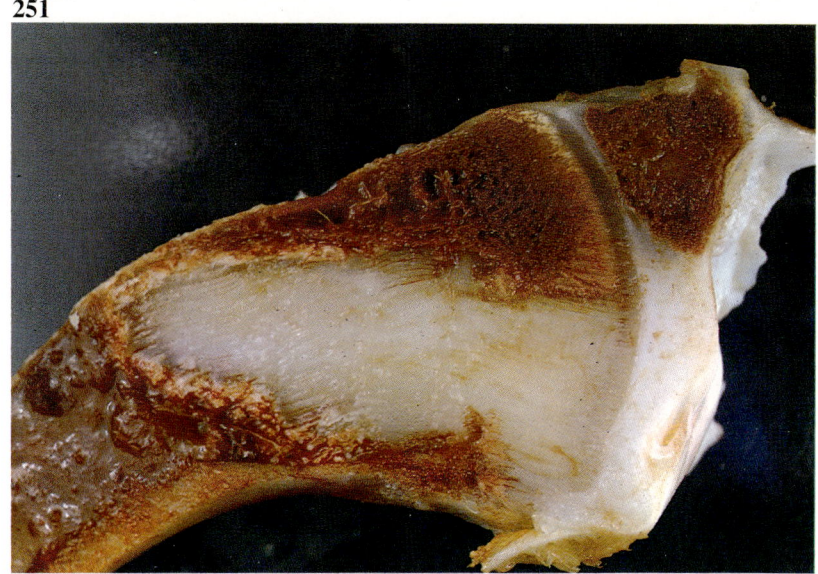

252

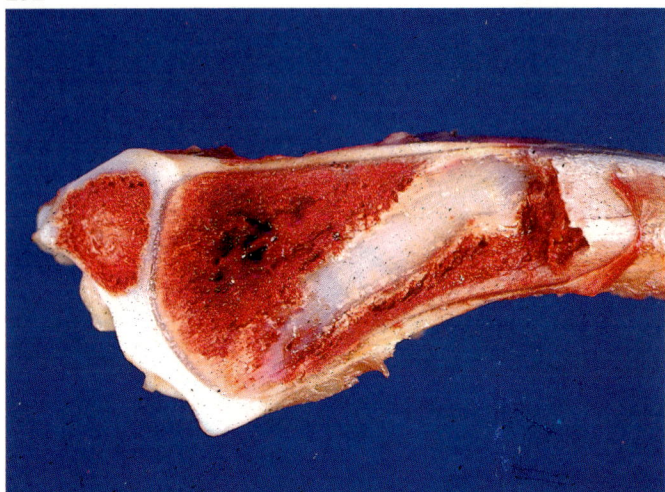

253

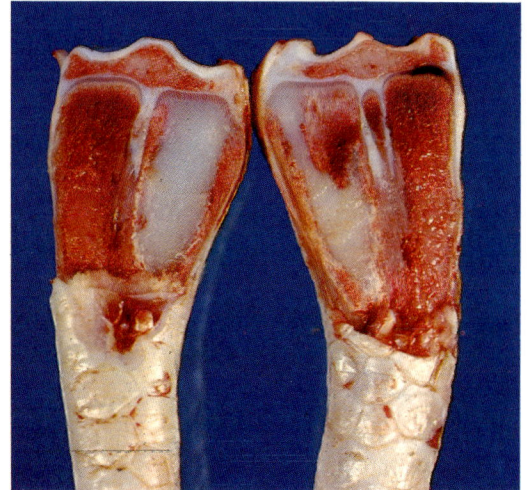

254

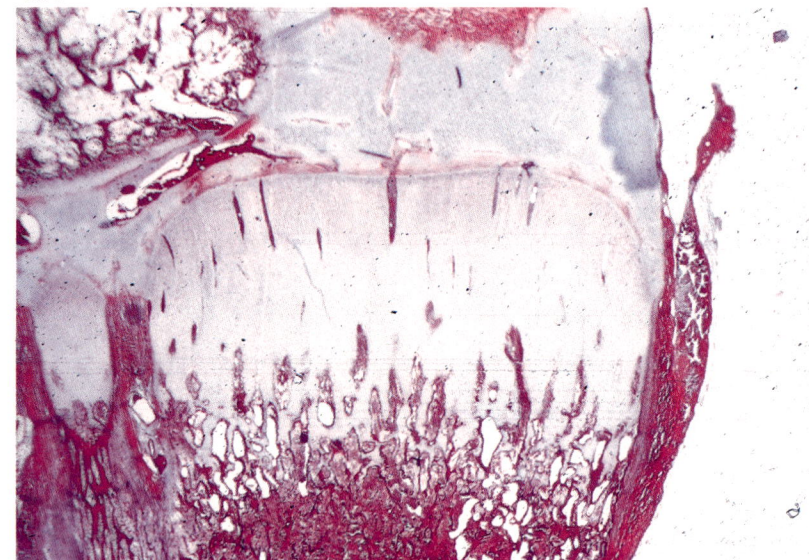

252 The lesion has been partially re-
solved in this bone but a substantial
quantity of abnormal cartilage still
remains.

253 Varus deformity of tarsometatarsi associated with large medial
plugs of cartilage in a broiler of
slaughter age. Many broilers are
affected by dyschondroplasia but do
not have deformed legs unless the
lesions are large.

254 Low power view of a shallow
dyschondroplastic lesion in the
proximal tarsometatarsus of a broiler.
Martius scarlet blue.

255 An area of abnormal cartilage in
the metaphysis. The metaphyseal
blood vessels are numerous but those
near the periphery of the hypertrophic
cartilage appear empty (arrows) and
hardly invade the cartilage. Martius
scarlet blue.

255

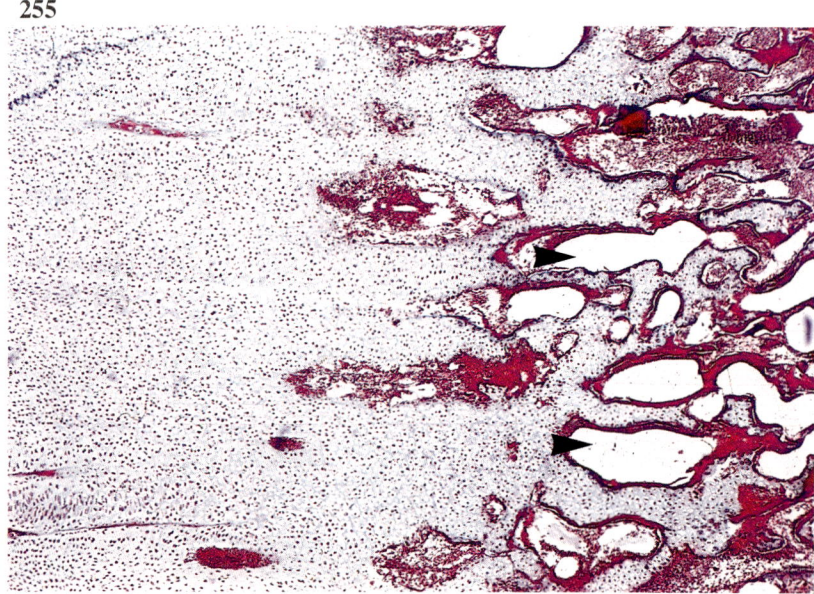

256 The lack of blood supply to the hypertrophic cartilage leads to necrosis of the distal cells. Necrotic cartilage cells containing eosinophilically staining nuclei are scattered amongst other surviving cells.

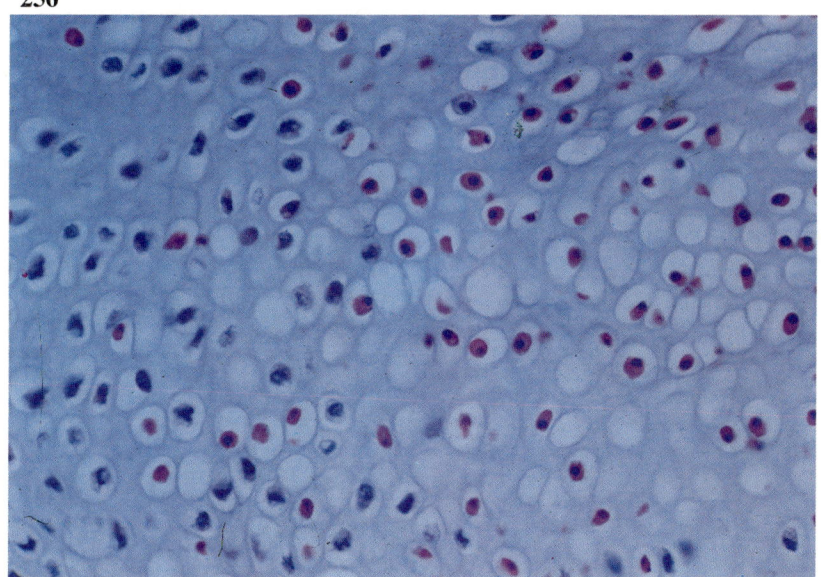

Valgus leg deformity in broilers ('twisted leg')

257 Valgus deformity is seen from two weeks of age onwards and may affect either one or both legs. Males are more often affected than females. Affected legs bend outwards at the hock joint. Posterior aspect.

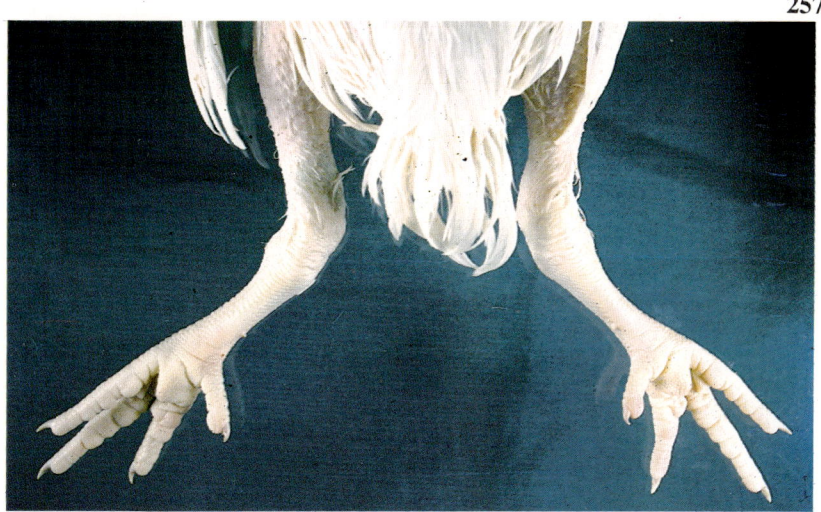

258 Removal of the musculature shows that in most cases the deformity results from a lateral tilting (rather than twisting) of the distal tibiotarsal condyles. Anterior aspect.

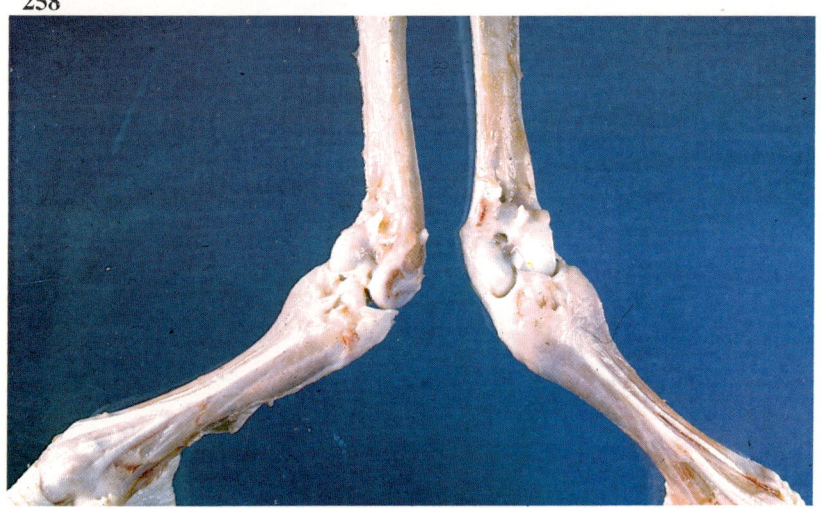

259 Progressively severe deformity affecting three legs from left to right. As the condition becomes more severe the gastrocnemius tendon slips off the joint and usually comes to lie laterally over the bone. Anterior aspect.

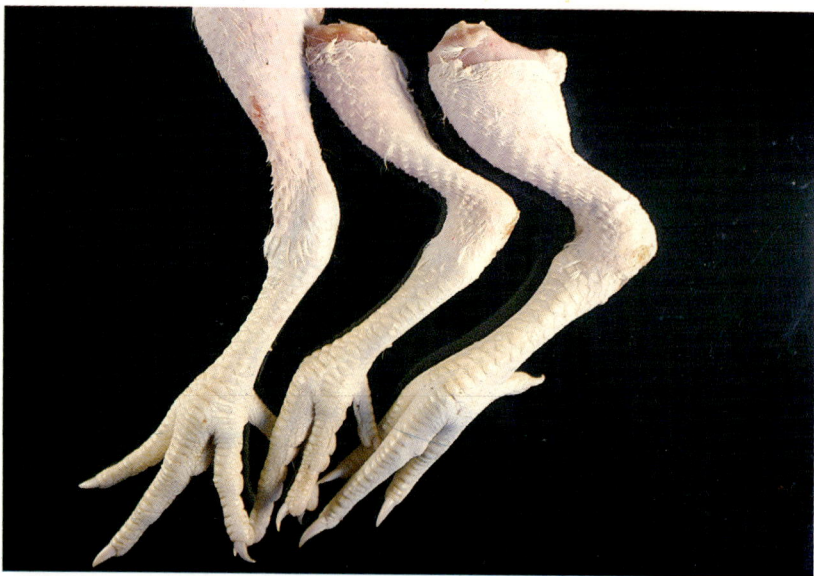

260 The lateral deviation of the distal tibiotarsal condyles may be sufficiently severe for them to become separated from the shaft of the bone. In this broiler the shaft has come to lie underneath the skin just above the hock joint.

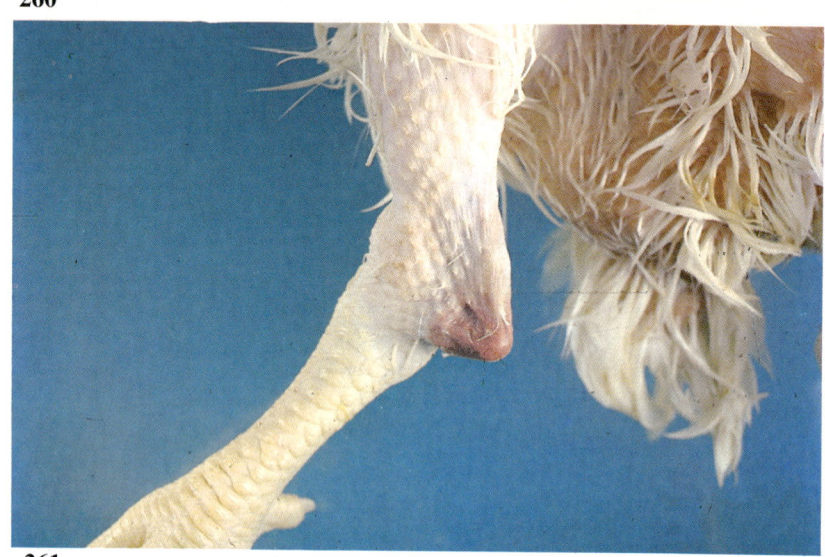

261 A dissected hock joint of a broiler shows the condyles at right angles to the shaft of the bone. Dyschondroplasia may be found in the distal tibiotarsus of some severely deformed cases.

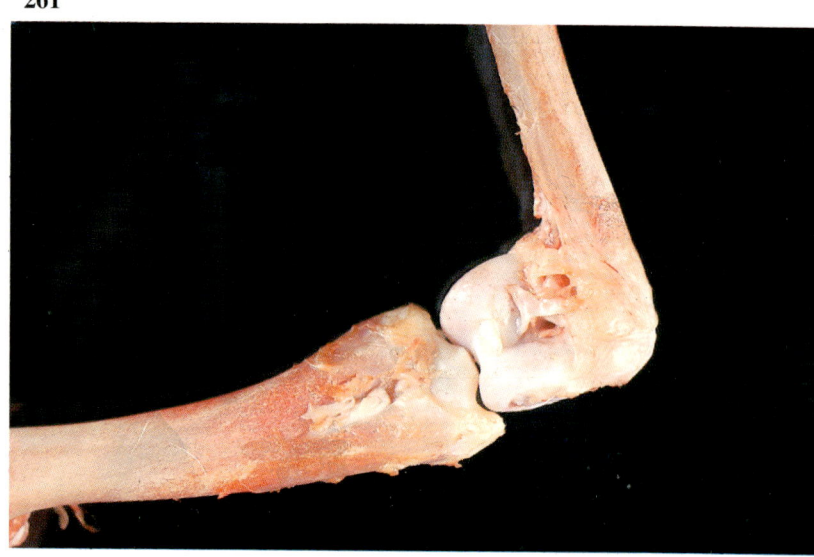

Twisted leg in turkeys

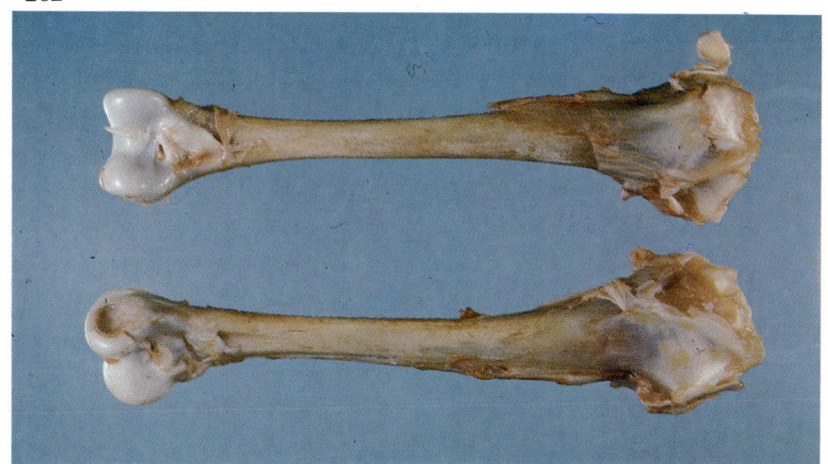

262 The lower third of the bottom tibiotarsus has rotated laterally. This process produces a similar overall effect to valgus deformity of the legs in broilers ('twisted leg'), but is usually restricted to one leg and is a true rotation of the shaft. It is occasionally seen in broilers.

Renal failure (visceral gout)

Renal failure is a common cause of death in fowls of different types and ages. It is also seen in the turkey. Apart from recognised causes of renal disease such as nephritis induced by infectious bronchitis virus, water deprivation, and excessive intake of protein and calcium the aetiology of many of the nephritides and nephroses is uncertain. Visceral gout, *ie* the deposition of urates on the surfaces of the viscera and in the joints, should not be regarded as a single entity but as an end stage of possibly many different renal diseases. Generally, kidney disease is more prevalent in adult laying fowl.

263 Baby chick nephropathy may occur during the first week of life and cause heavy mortality. Birds may die shortly after hatching. The kidneys are swollen and urates are usually deposited on the viscera and in the joints (visceral gout). Histologically, there may be scattered foci of necrotic tissue throughout the cortex or dilation and inflammation of the collecting duct system and ureteral branches.

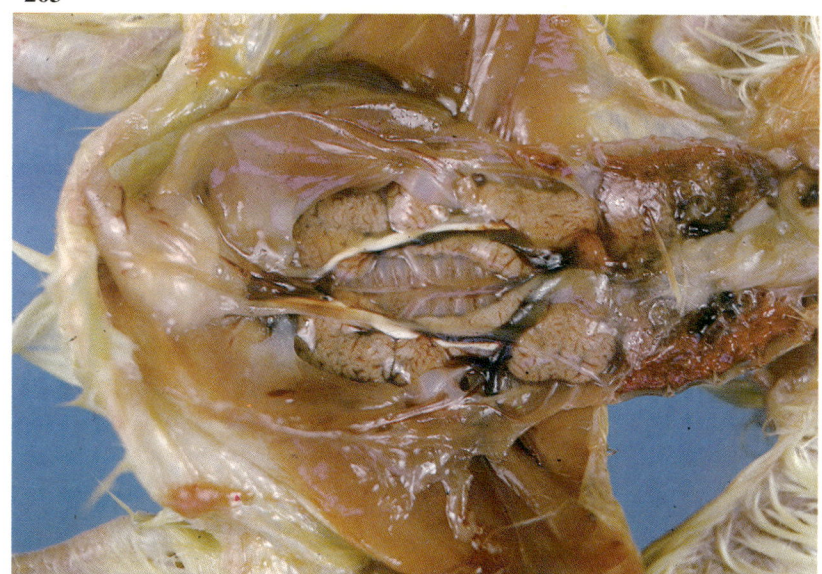

264 Urolithiasis. This condition has become more prevalent in laying fowl. Affected birds usually remain in lay until shortly before death. The carcases are congested. One or both kidneys show signs of atrophy. The ureters are greatly distended with mucus and uroliths.

264

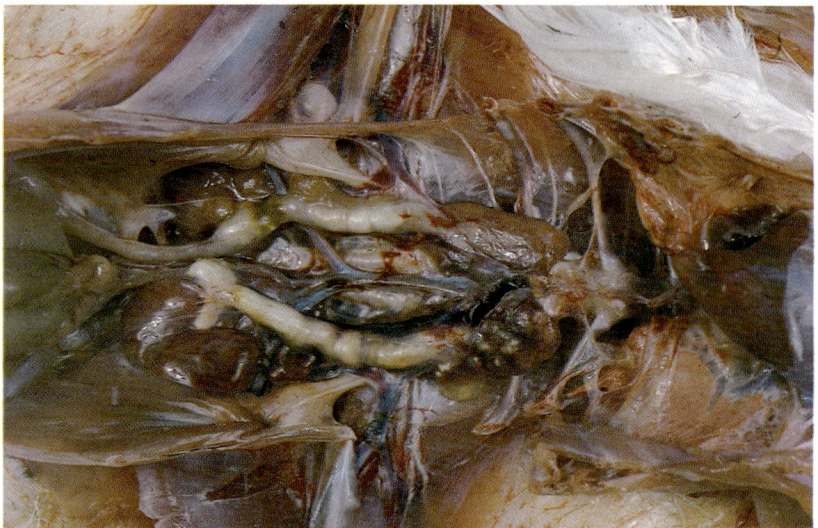

265 Urolithiasis. This adult broiler breeder hen died in good bodily condition. One kidney has almost completely atrophied. Compensatory hypertrophy has taken place in the divisions of the opposite organ which is drained by a large distended ureter (arrows). Urates are present on the surface of the epicardium.

265

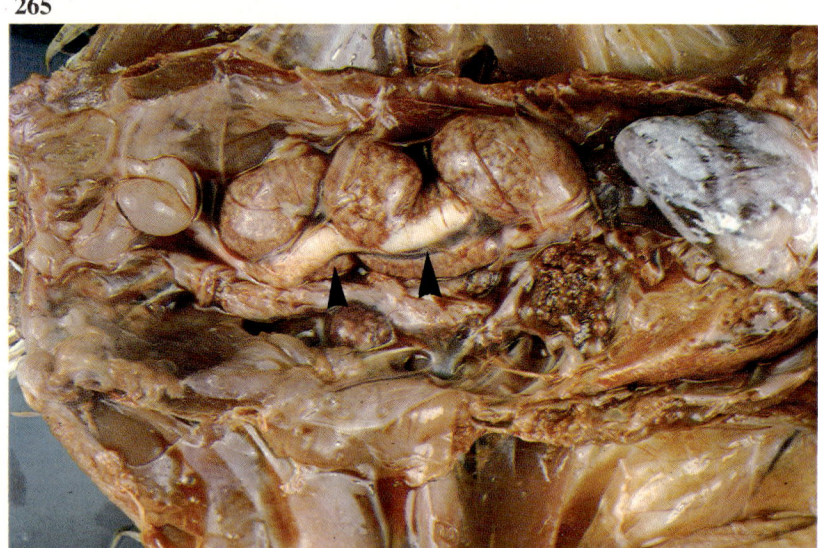

266 Urolithiasis. A greatly distended ureter on the left almost obscured the atrophic kidney on that side. Compensatory hypertrophy has taken place on the right. These kidneys were dissected from an adult commercial layer.

266

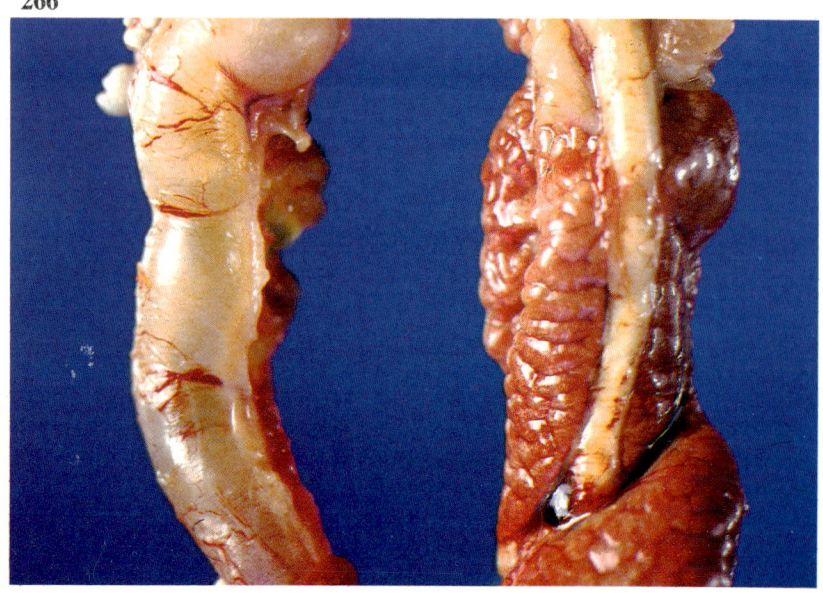

267 Urolithiasis. Dilated collecting tubules in a medullary tract of an adult laying fowl. Masses of inflammatory cells are present within the tubules. There is usually an interstitial nephritis.

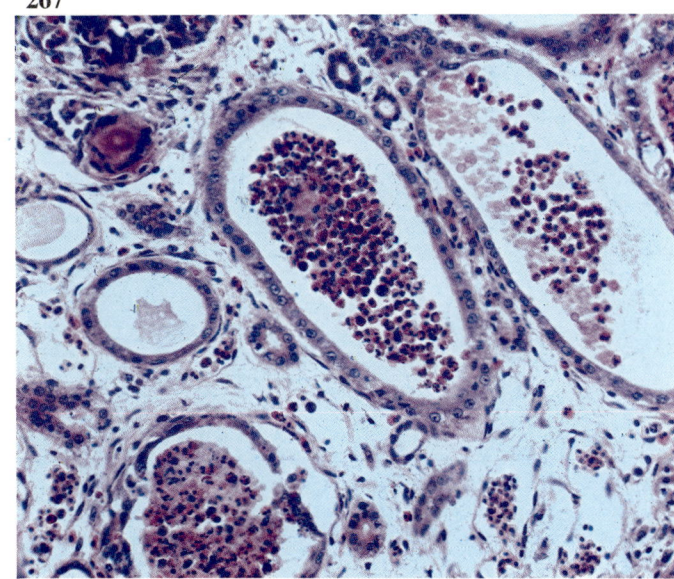

268 Urolithiasis. A focal area of necrosis within the cortex, probably resulting from coalescing degenerate proximal convoluted tubules. Note dilation of the surrounding tubules and flattening of their epithelium.

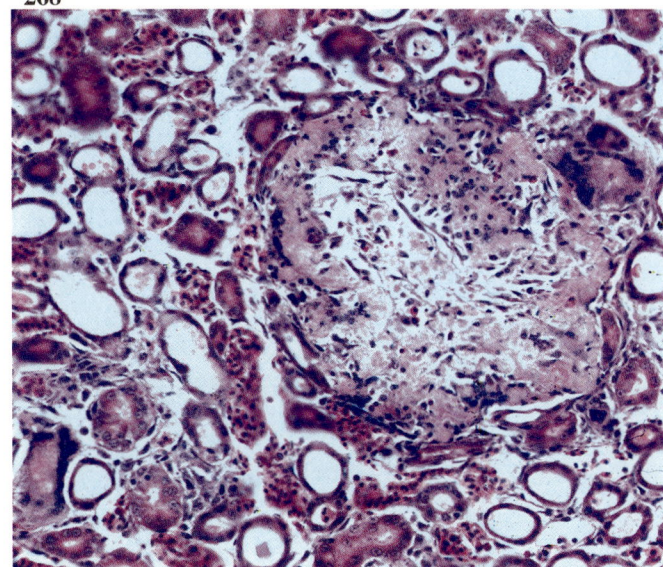

269 The cross-section of the kidney on the right emphasis the considerable size that hypertrophied renal divisions may attain. The tissue on the left of the photograph, although fairly autolysed, demonstrates the size of the corresponding division in a normal kidney obtained from a bird of similar age.

270 Visceral gout. Deposition of urates on the epicardium.

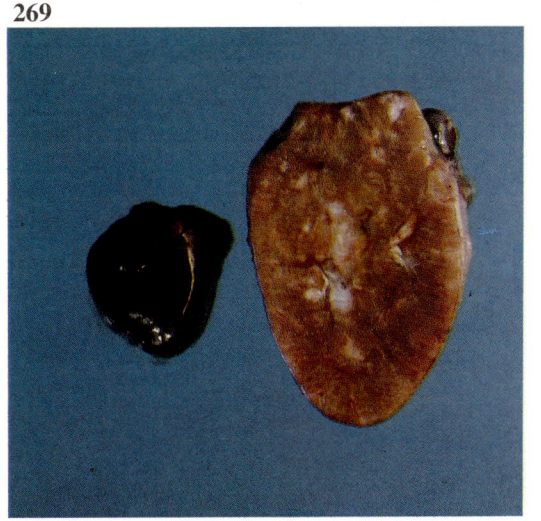

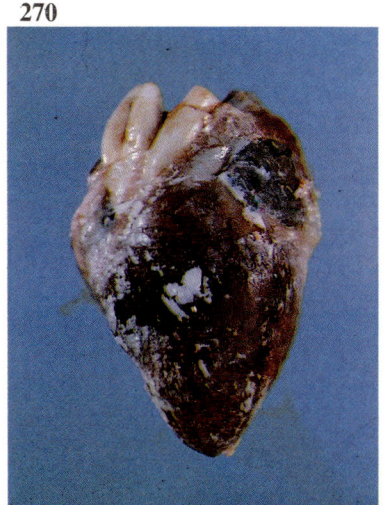

271 Visceral gout. Urates contained within a hock joint.

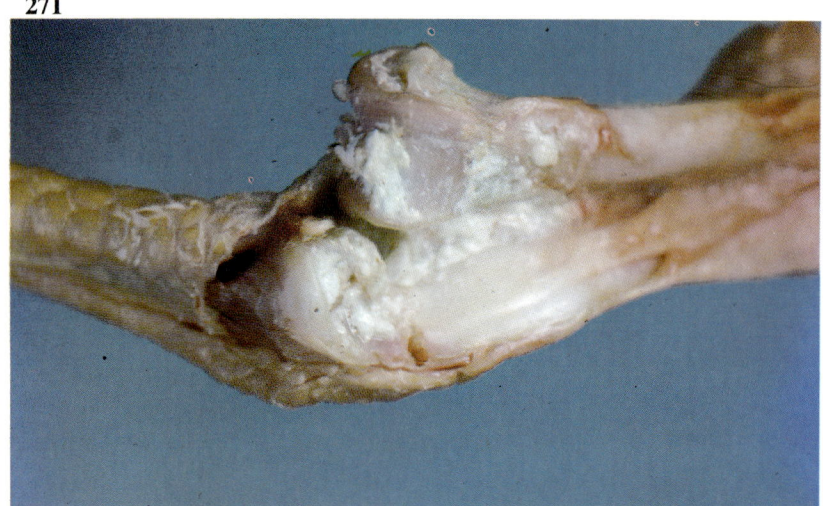

272 Visceral gout. Urates present on the surface of the liver, abdominal fat and sternum.

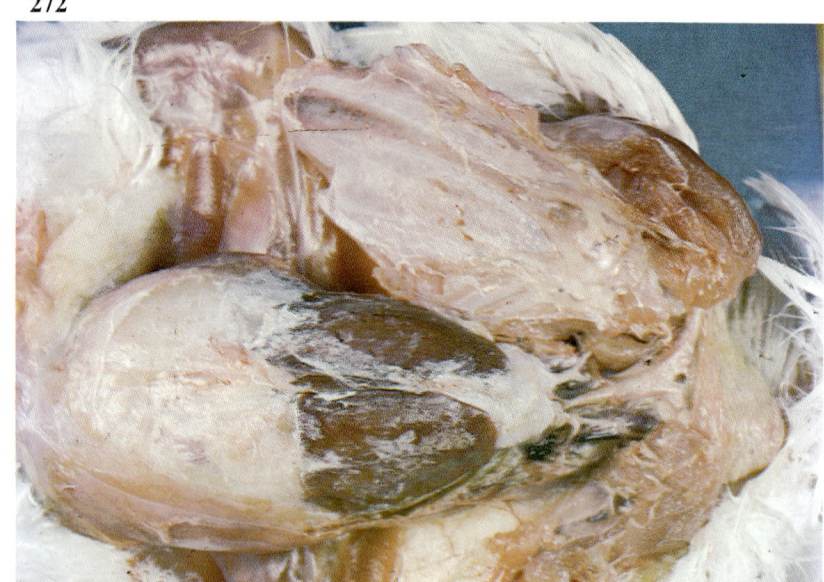

273 Articular gout. Periarticular deposition of urates in two feet. Normal foot on the right for comparison.

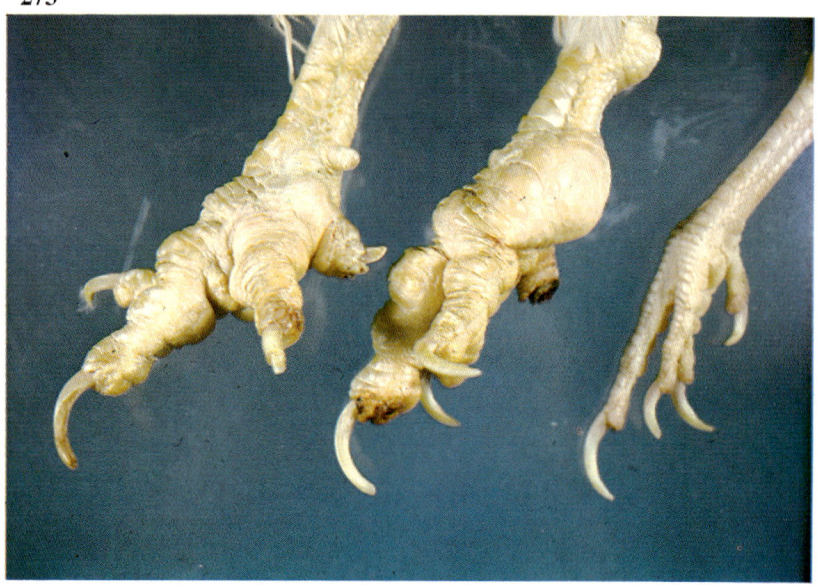

274 Visceral gout. Tophus formation may occur terminally in the kidney and other tissues such as the liver and spleen. In this renal focus the urates have dissolved out of the tissue during processing but the radial pattern of their deposition is still visible.

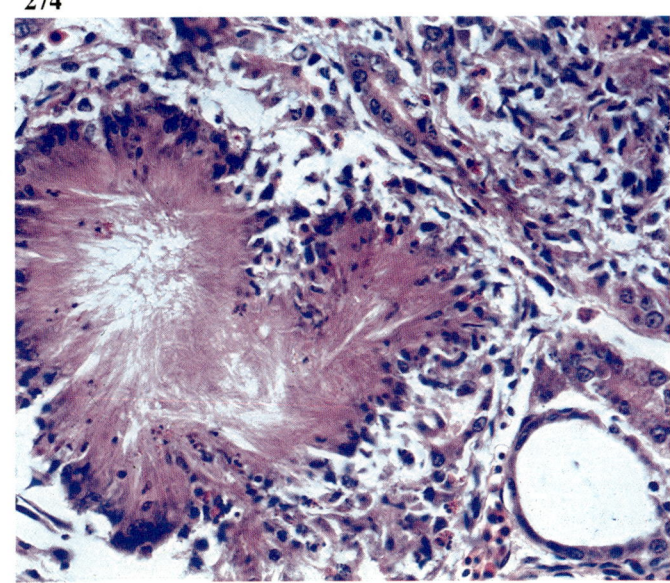

275 Visceral gout. Tophus formation within the cortex (tissue fixed in absolute alcohol and stained by the Gomori methenamine silver method).

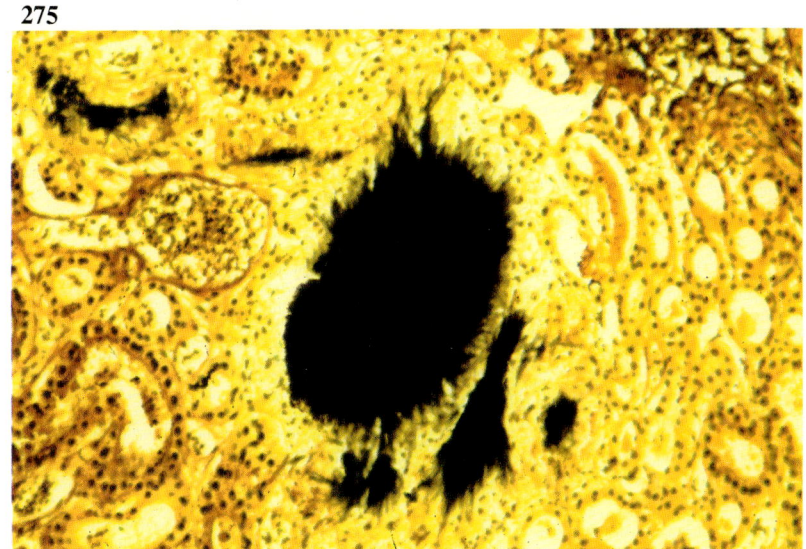

Stunting syndrome of broilers (malabsorption)

276 This is a transmissible condition which becomes most noticeable clinically during the second week of life. Both of the birds shown are 23 days of age. Note the retention of chick down on the small bird and also the abdominal protrusion. Abnormalities of the primary wing feathers may result in a "helicopter" appearance.

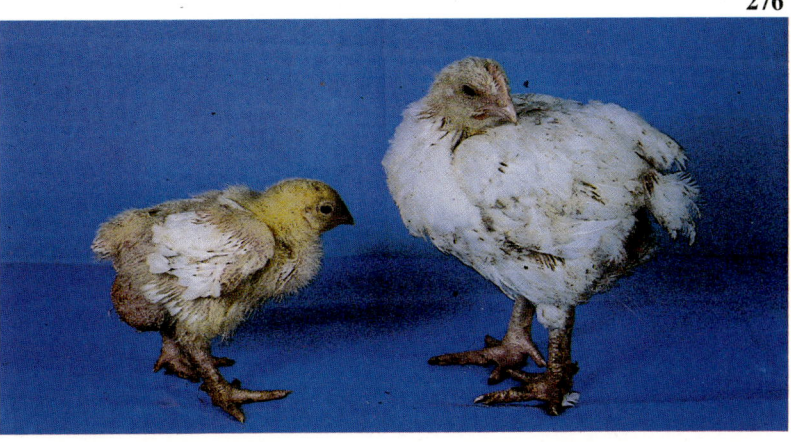

277 Gross lesions vary in different outbreaks. One of the features of the disease in Britain has been the appearance of pancreatic lesions. A pale fibrosed pancreas (bottom) in a stunted 5-week-old broiler is compared with the normal gland in a 3-week-old specimen from the same farm. Pancreatic tissue at the closed end of the duodenal loop is usually affected first.

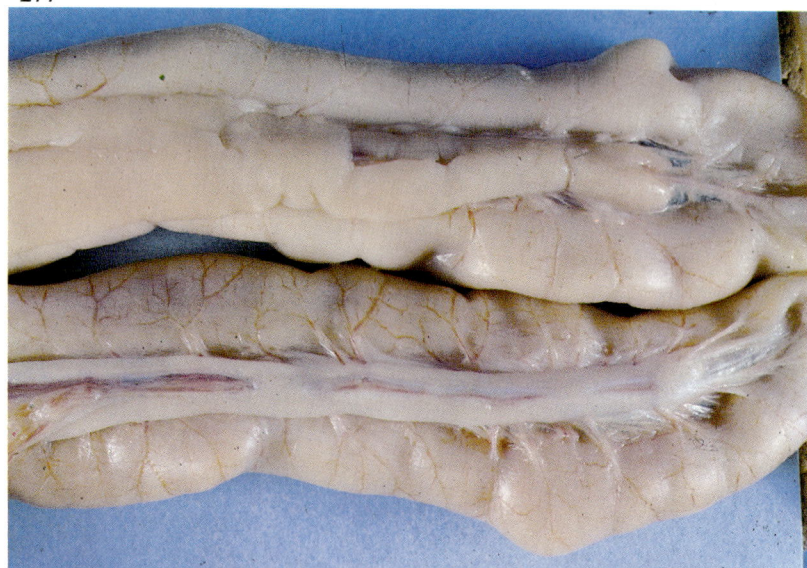

278 The lesions are mainly confined to the exocrine pancreas. Early stages of degeneration, atrophy and fibrosis are taking place. There is considerable vacuolation of the acinar cells and only a few of these contain zymogen granules. Acrylic resin.

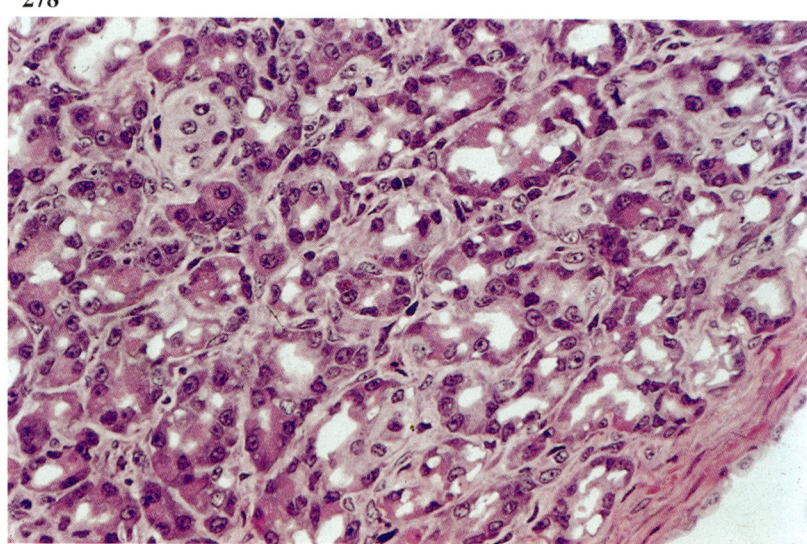

279 High power view of the abnormal pancreas. The acinar cells on the right contain zymogen granules but these are absent in the tissue on the left. Acrylic resin, haematoxylin ponceau fuschin.

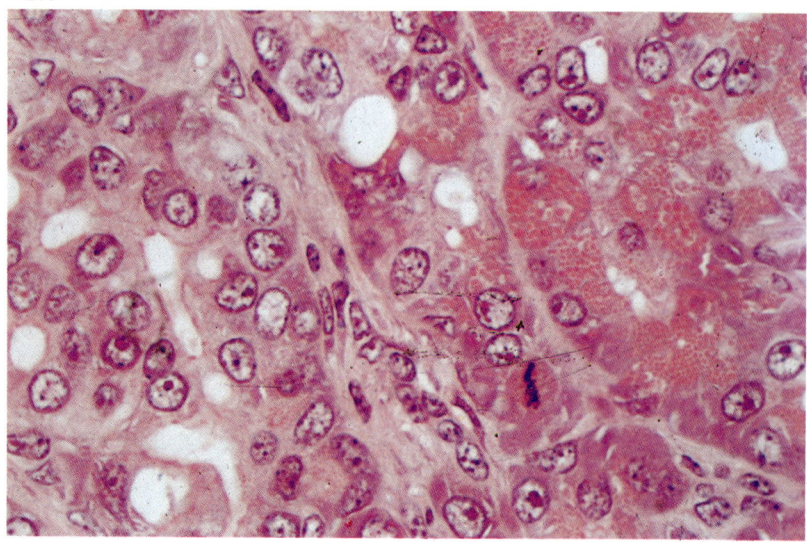

280 Side view of the distended abdomen in a 2-week-old broiler.

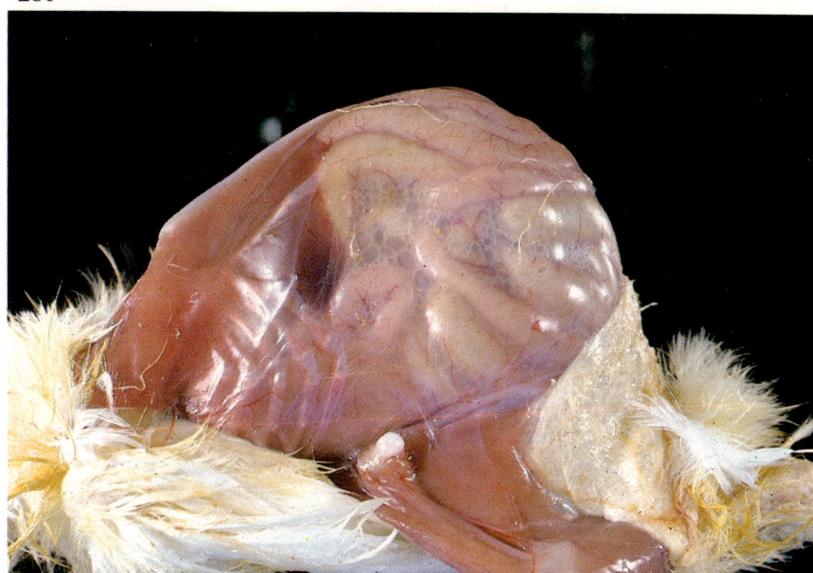

281 The intestines are pale and dilated, this dilation giving rise to the abdominal distension. Undigested food is present in the lower bowel. The pale pancreas (arrow) can be seen in the duodenal loop.

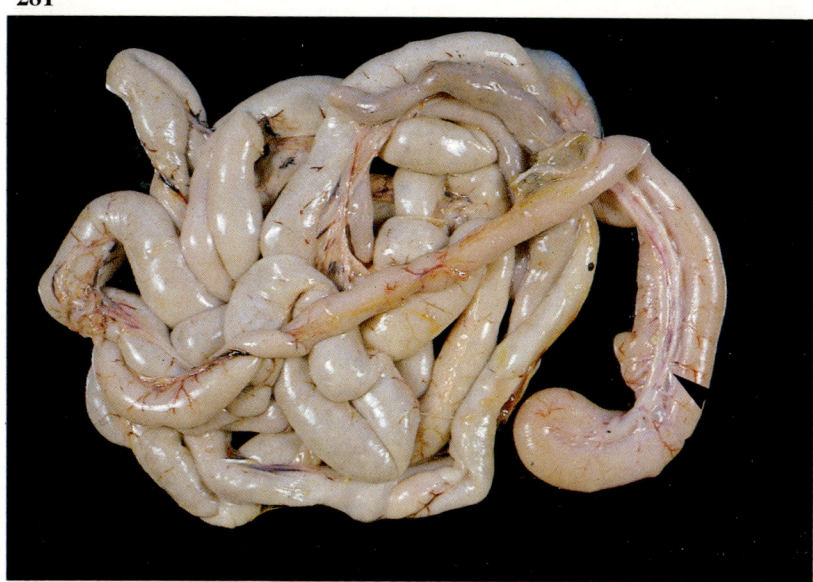

282 Proventricular swelling has been a less common finding in Britain.

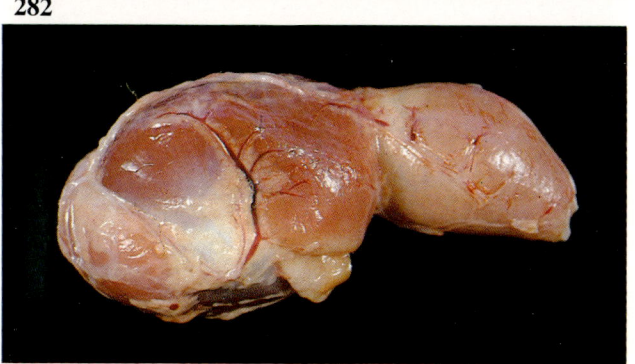

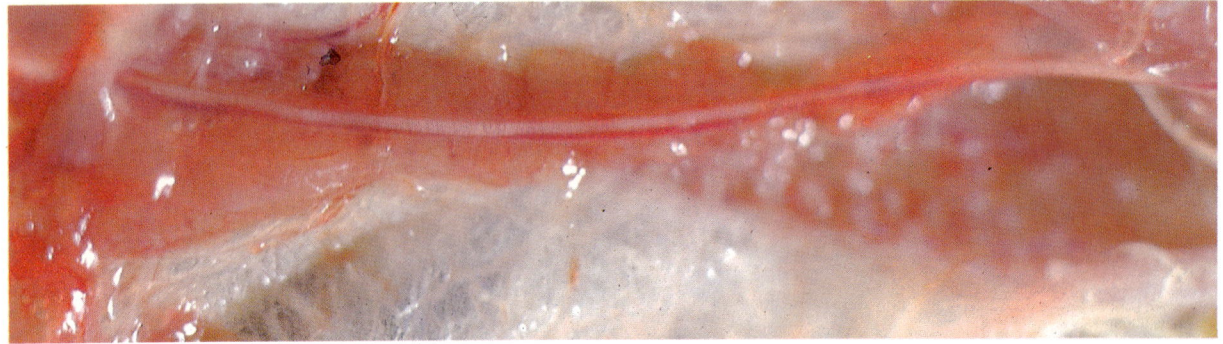

283 Atrophy of thymus in a 3-week-old broiler. The vagal nerve is lying dorsally to small reddened portions of gland.

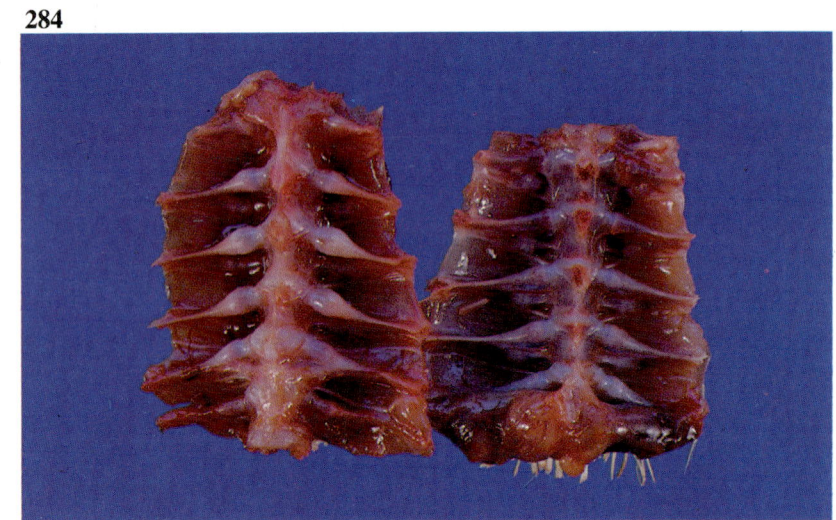

284 Rickety changes may affect the skeleton. Note swollen rib heads from a stunted broiler on the left compared to a normal specimen (*see* **208**).

Acute pectoral myopathy of broiler breeders

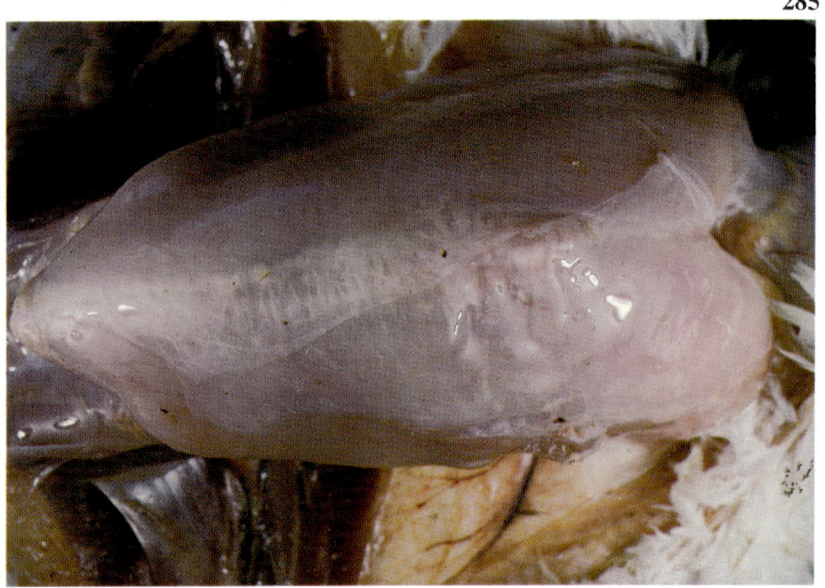

285 A sporadically occurring condition in immature birds during the rearing period. Affected birds are not usually seen ill. Gelatinous fluid is often present in the subcutaneous tissue overlying the breast and also separates muscle fibre groups within the *Musculus pectoralis*. Pools of this fluid may collect between the *M. pectoralis* and the *M. supracoracoideus*.

286 Severe myodegeneration in a *M. pectoralis*. Masson's trichrome.

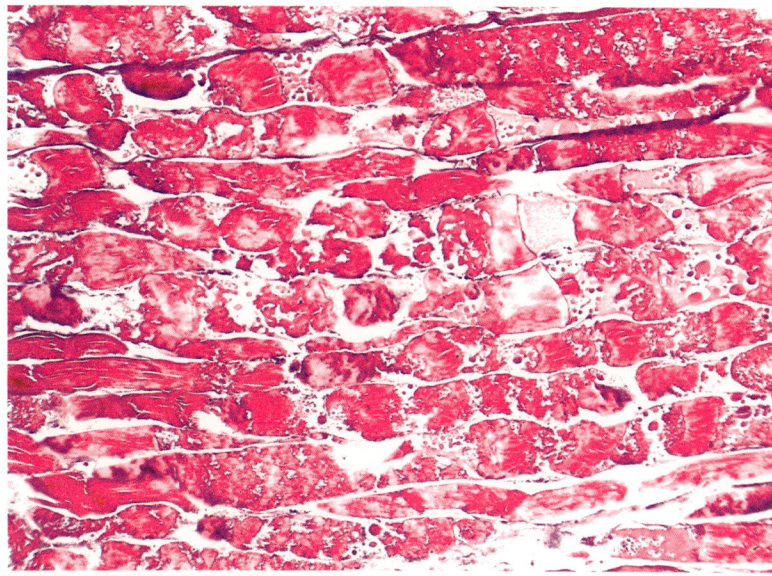

287 Contraction of necrotic segments of cytoplasm in three fibres of the *M. pectoralis*. Note the pale blue staining fluid filling the emptied portions of the endomysial tubes. Masson's trichrome.

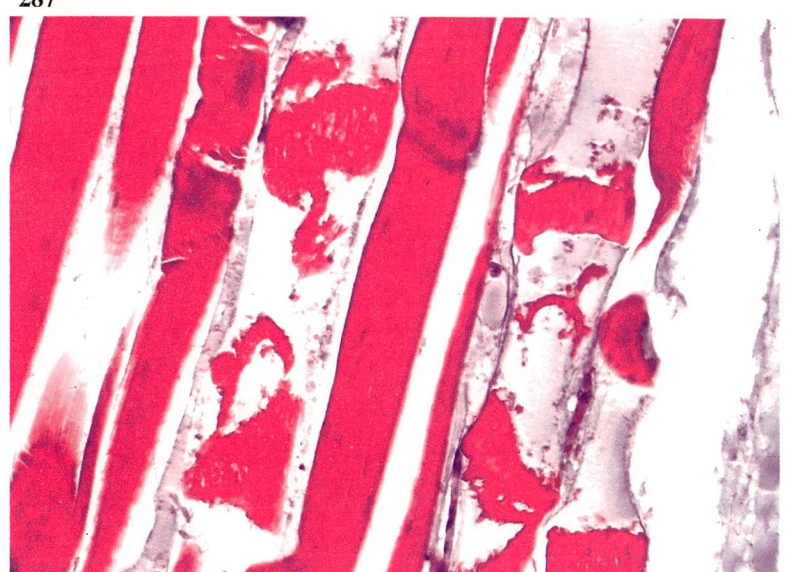

Miscellaneous conditions

Spondylolisthesis (kinky back)

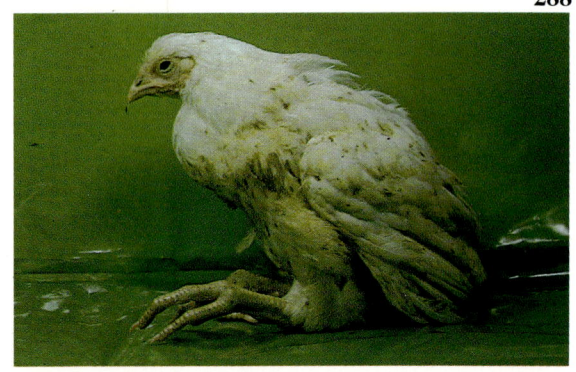

288 Clinical cases are usually seen in broilers between 3 and 6 weeks of age. Birds squat back on their hocks and cannot stand. One or both feet are often slightly raised from the surface on which they are placed.

289 The condition is caused by a downward rotation of the sixth thoracic vertebral body. If sufficiently severe, this results in a failure of the interarticular facets between the sixth and seventh thoracic vertebrae with the result that the sixth vertebra moves ventrally and compresses the spinal cord (arrow).

289

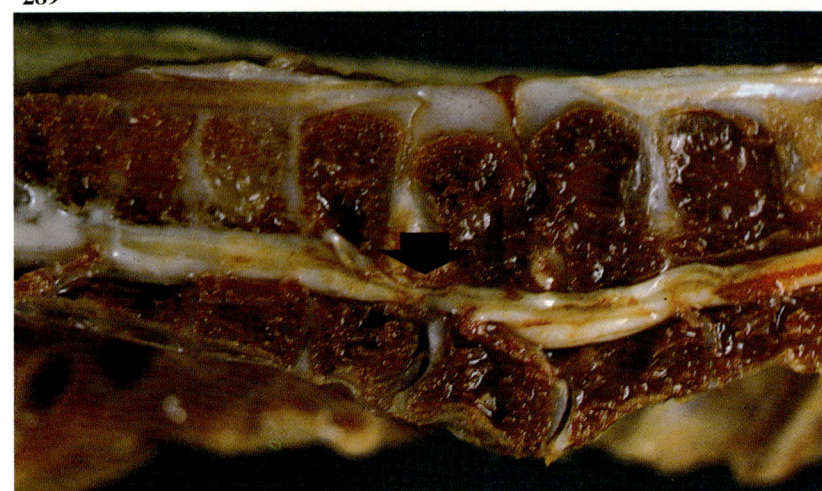

290 Spinal cord with compressed zone (arrow).

290

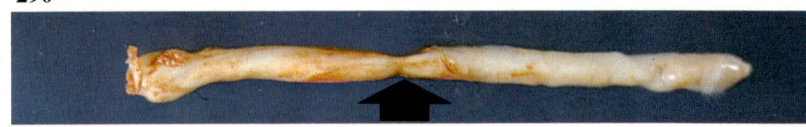

291 Section of spinal column at T6/T7 showing compression of spinal cord.

291

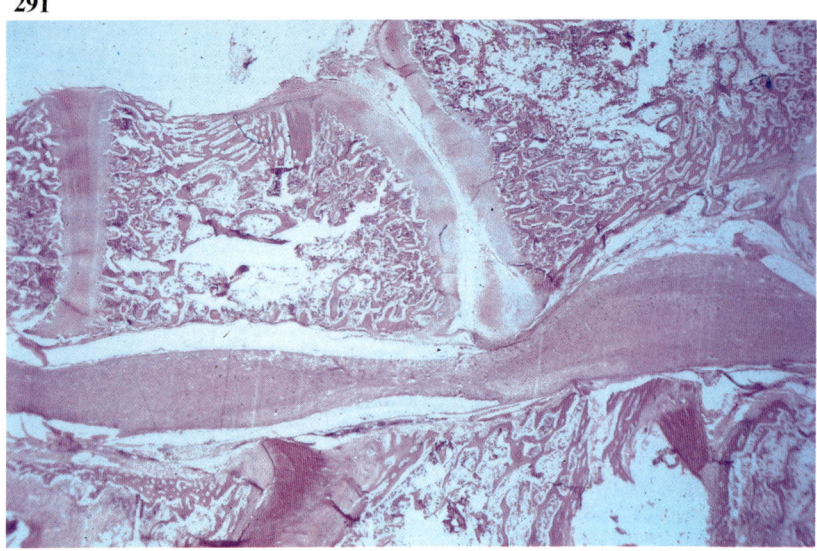

Ruptured gastrocnemius tendon

292 This may occur sporadically, usually in heavy fowl such as capons and broiler breeders, but is occasionally seen as an outbreak. The condition may be uni- or bilateral. Viral arthritis should be suspected if the rupture has been preceded by a chronic tendinitis and tenosynovitis (*see* **120-123**).

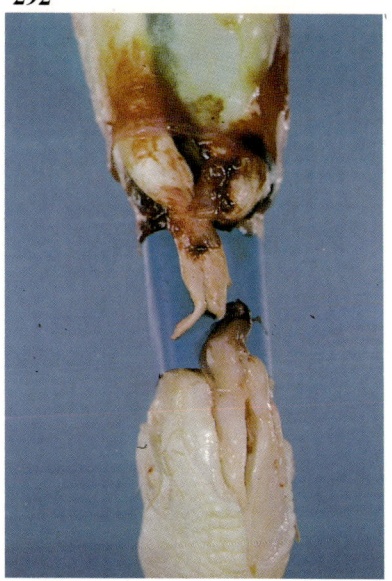

Deep pectoral myopathy

293 Occurs in turkeys and broiler breeders. The condition is usually observed at meat inspection. The lesion may affect either one or both of the deep pectoral muscles (*M. supracoracoideus*). This turkey breeder carcase has dished pectoral musculature on the right of the photograph. A black line has been drawn over the breast to distinguish the two sides.

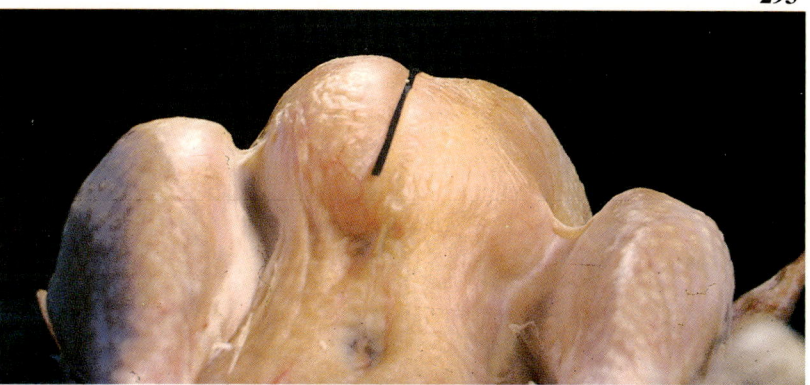

294 The *M. supracoracoideus* is contained in an osteofascial compartment. Abnormal exercise for birds of this type such as undue flapping of wings may in some individuals lead to swelling of the muscle and occlusion of its blood supply. Necrosis results. The fascia of the muscle of this 33-week-old broiler breeder has been cut anteriorly to show the bulging affected tissue (arrows) of the acute lesion. The early lesion is accompanied by the production of gelatinous fluid.

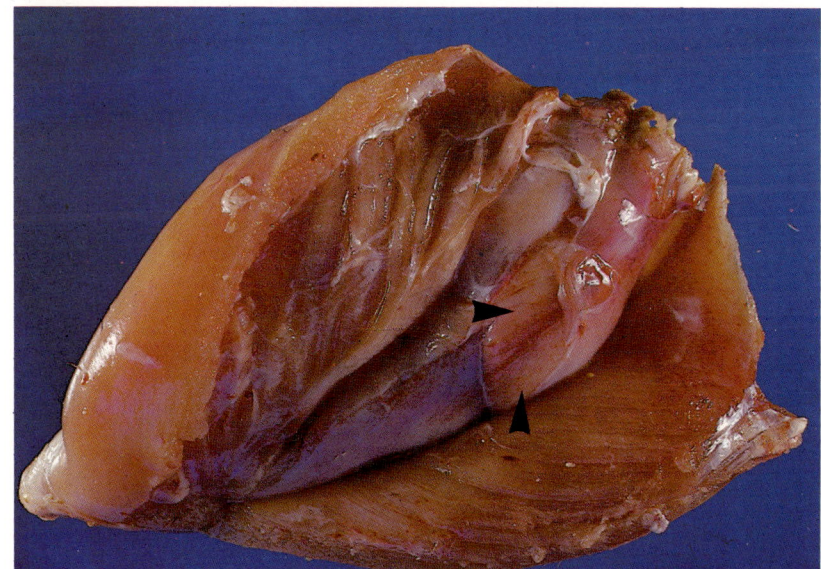

295 The bottom muscle is an affected *M. supracoracoideus* that is undergoing atrophy. The necrotic tissue is often an unusual apple green colour. The medio-ventral aspect is shown.

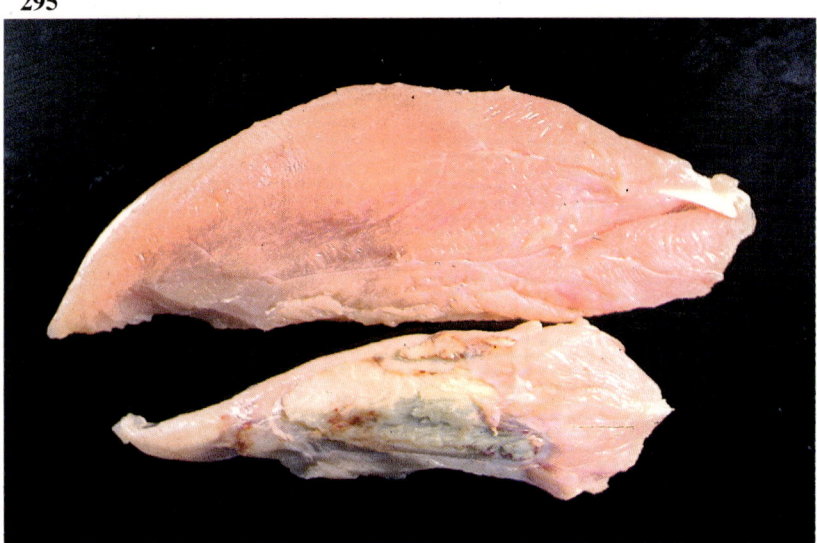

296 Cross section of affected and unaffected *M. supracoracoideus*. The necrotic tissue is crumbly and dry.

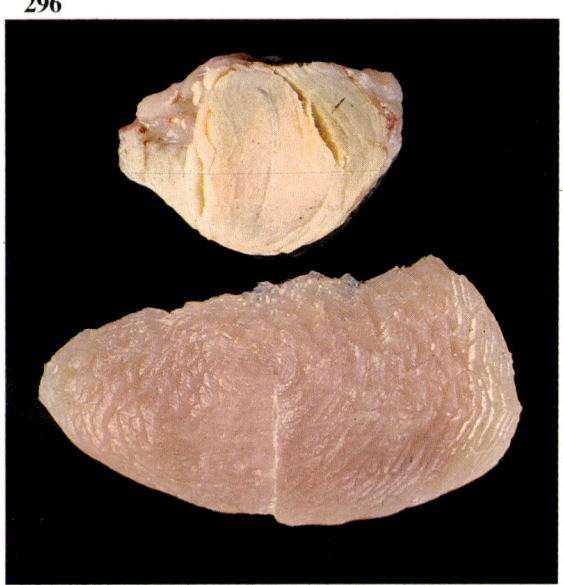

297 Cooked lesion. The green colour is retained.

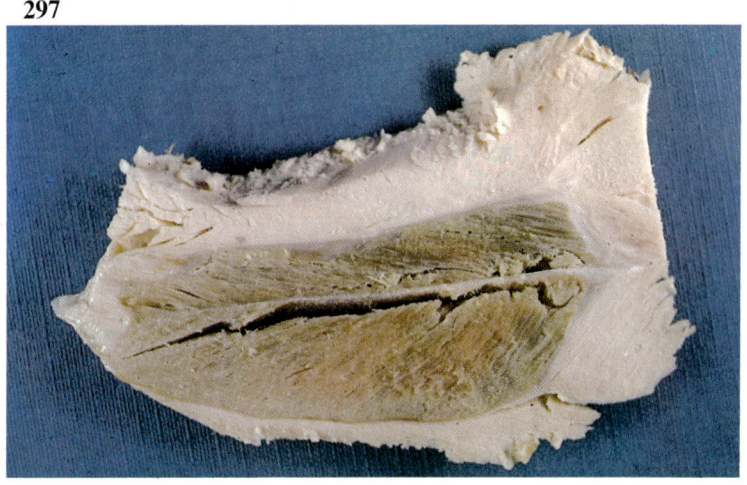

298 Fragments of necrotic *M. supra-coracoideus* (arrows) adhering to the sternum of a turkey breeder.

298

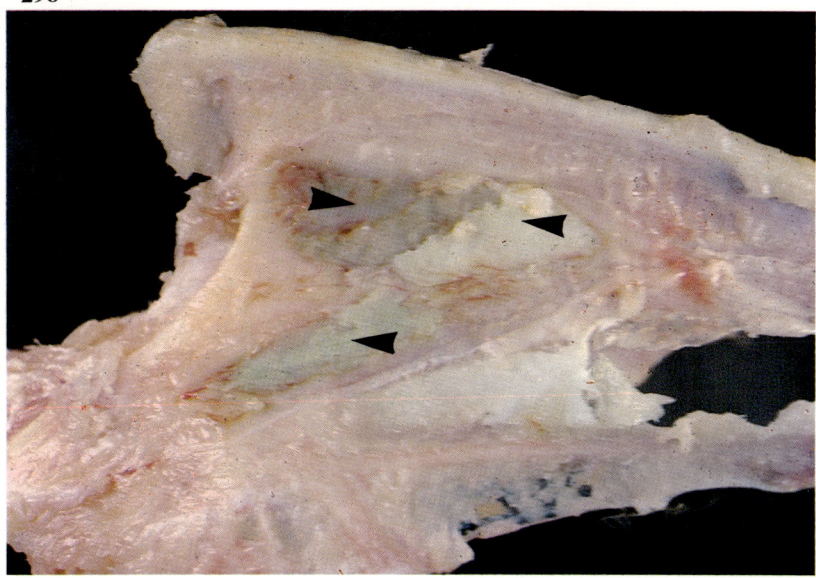

299 Junctions of normal and affected *M. supracoracoideus*. The necrotic tissue below is staining more palely with eosin than the viable muscle above.

299

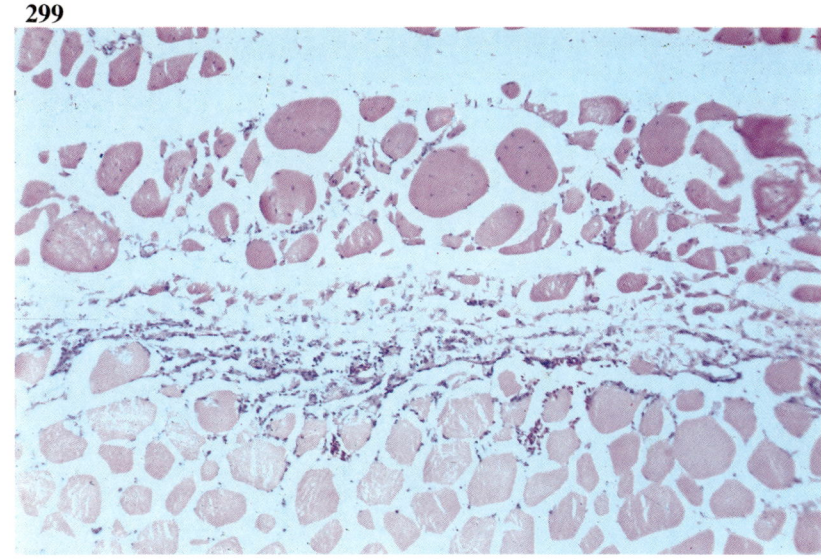

300 Muscle fibres within an affected *M. supracoracoideus*. These exhibit discoid necrosis.

300

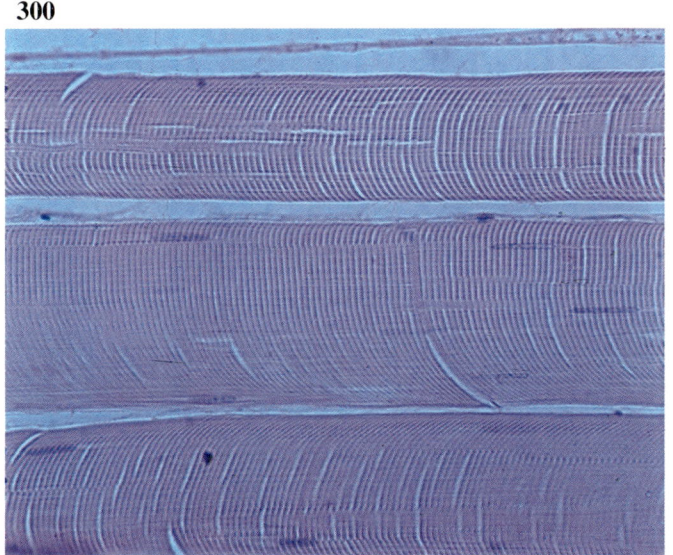

Plantar pododermatitis

301 The plantar surface of the foot-pads of heavy broiler breeders and turkeys may become severely ulcerated and caked with litter. This is seen most frequently when the litter conditions are poor, particularly if flocks are scouring.

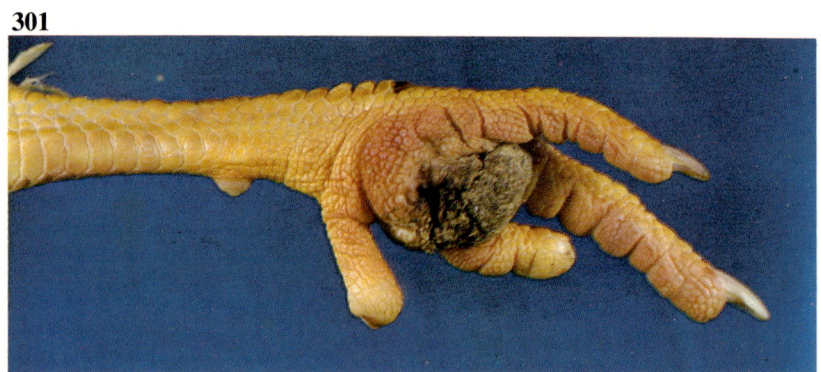

Moult

302 Although obviously not a disease, moult may be precipitated by events such as accidental water deprivation. A large number of new feathers are growing on the back of this broiler breeder.

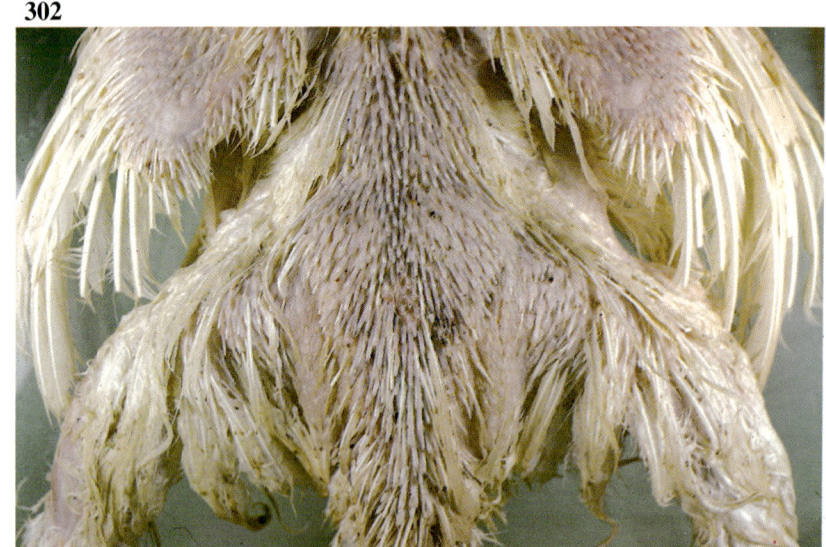

303 The ovaries of birds that are producing new feathers are inactive.

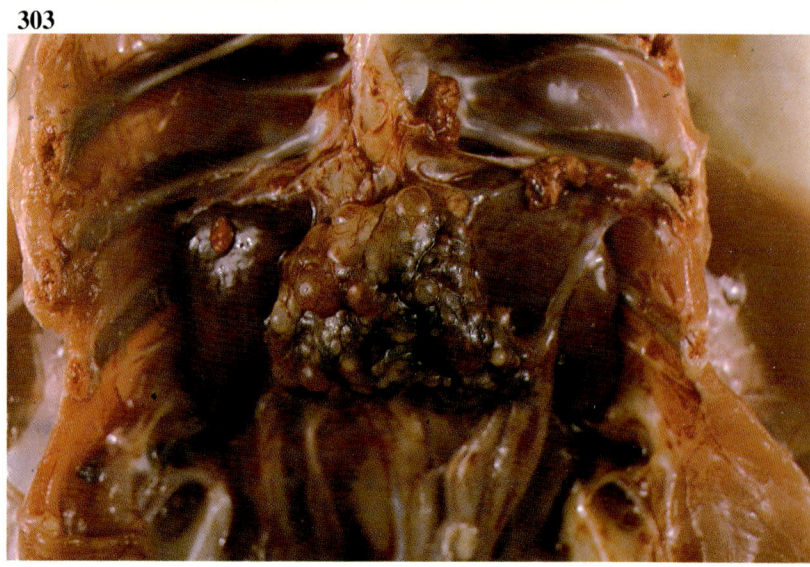

304 Moult must be distinguished from feather loss on the back as a result of mating activity in breeding flocks. Short stubby ends of broken feathers are usually apparent in these birds.

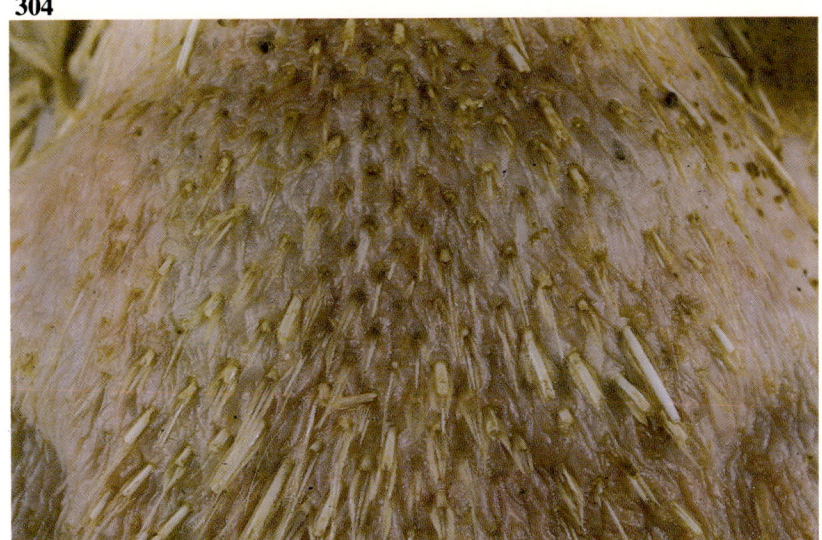

Persistent right oviduct

305 Cystic dilation of this structure (indicated by blue pointer) is a fairly common post-mortem finding. In some cases the cystic remnant may become very large and compress the abdominal viscera. Death can result.

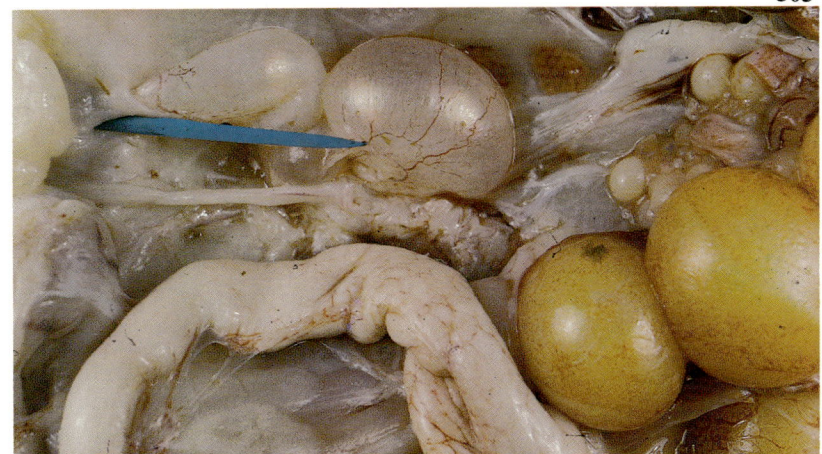

Internal layer

306 Three large soft shelled eggs were found in the abdomen of this commercial layer. The magnum was constricted at one point and had not permitted normal passage of eggs through the oviduct. Several more eggs are retained within the duct. Either soft or hard shelled eggs are occasionally found within the abdominal cavity of laying fowl that possess patent oviducts. These may be adherent to the peritoneum.

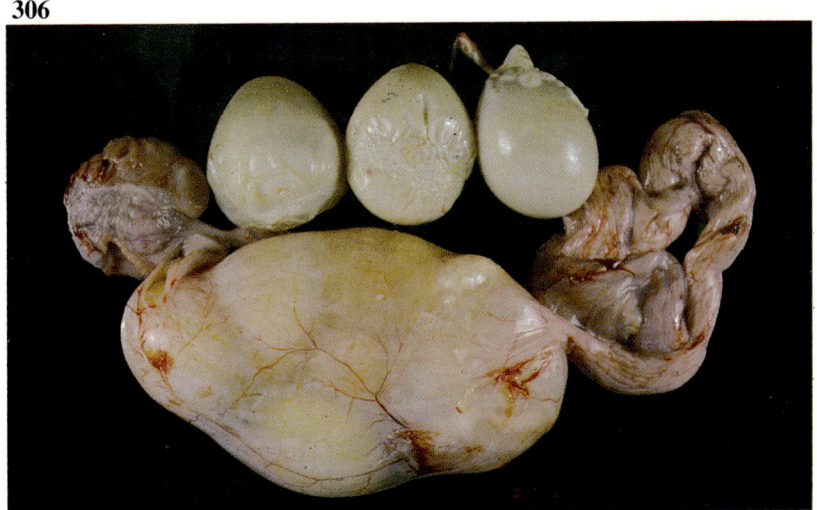

Prolapse of oviduct

307 The lower part of the oviduct is protruding through the vent.

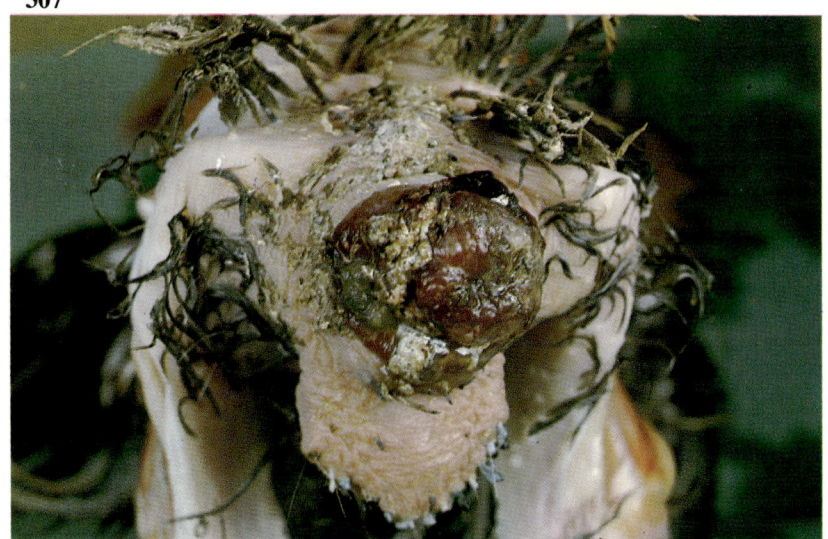

307

Cannibalism

308 In laying fowl the vent is most frequently attacked. At post-mortem examination most carcasses are pale and have usually part or all of the intestines and reproductive tract missing.

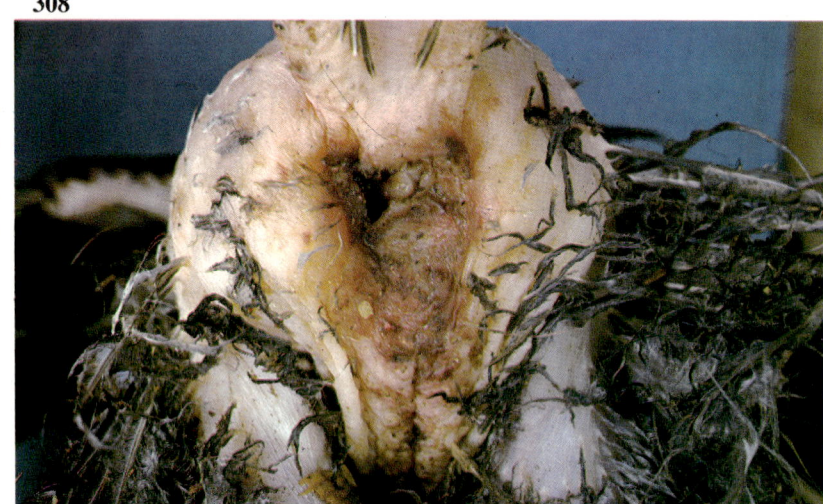

308

Poor thriving in chicks and poults

309 Failure to thrive as a result of adverse environmental conditions is a common cause of death at 5-7 days of age. The pectoral musculature is very thin in this chick.

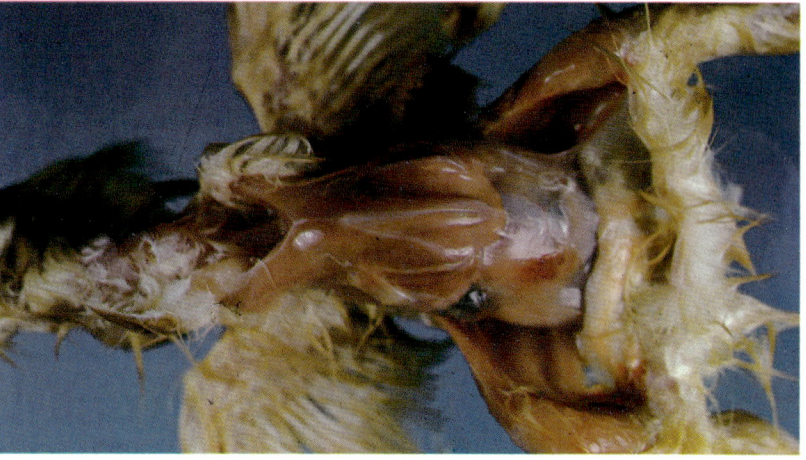

309

310 The gizzard is empty and stained with bile. An abnormally pale liver contains a distended gall bladder. Yolk sac absorption is usually advanced.

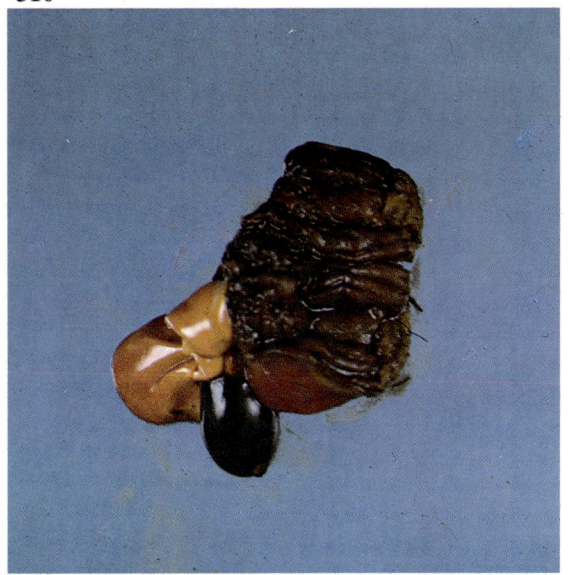

311 Although the quantity of fat within the liver of birds under one week of age is normally high, hepatic sections from specimens that have not thrived reveal an excessive amount of lipid. Oil red O.

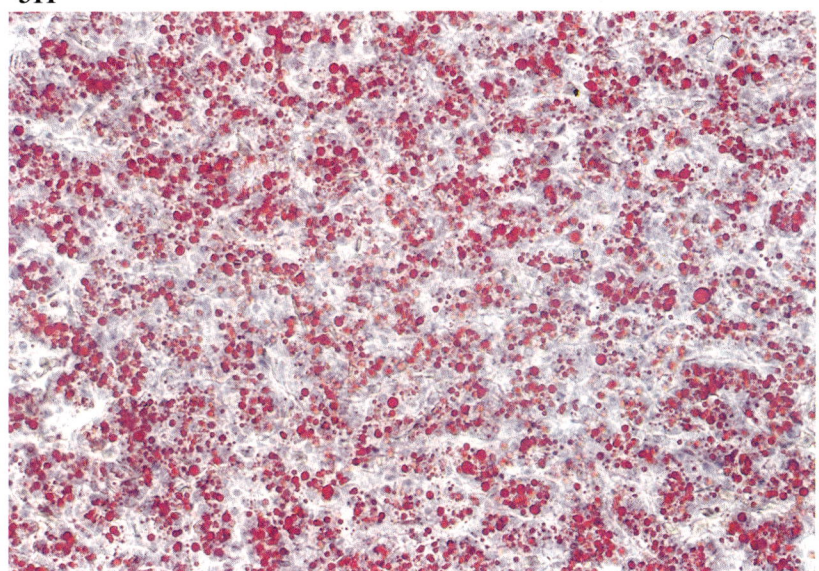

Selected reading

Coutts, G.S. (1981) *Poultry Diseases under Modern Management*, 2nd edition, Saiga Publishing.

Gordon, R.F. & Jordan, F.T.W. (Eds) (1982) *Poultry Diseases*, 2nd edition, Baillière Tindall.

Hofstad, M.S., Calnek, B.W., Helmboldt, C.F., Reid, W.M. & Yoder, H.W. (Eds) (1978) *Diseases of Poultry*, 7th edition, Iowa State University Press.

Index

References in this index are to Figure numbers.

Myelocytes, proliferating, myeloid leukosis, 148
Myelocytoma, myeloid leukosis, 147
Myeloid leukosis, 148-149
Myocarditis, listeriosis, 47
Myocardium, fat droplets, 224
Myopathy, acute pectoral, 285-287; deep pectoral, 293-300

Neck, cellulitis, 13; paralysis, 138
Necrosis, kidney, renal failure, 268; liver, salmonellosis, 60;
    liver, staphylococcal infection, 33-34; lung, gangrenous
    dermatitis, 46, lung, salmonellosis, 65; muscle, pectoral
    myopathy, 294-300, 293-300; mucosa, small intestine,
    coccidiosis, 189; necrotic enteritis 36-40
Necrotic enteritis, 36-42
Neoplasia, 126-136, 140-152, 153-156, 157
Nephritis, 109-110, 263, 267
Nephroblastoma, 151-152
Nephron dilation, necrotic enteritis, 41
Nerve, brachial, enlarged, 126; sciatic, normal, 125; sciatic,
    Schwann cell proliferation, 201
Neuron, brain stem, central chromatolysis, 116
Newcastle disease, 102-106, 115
Nodules, air sacs, aspergillosis, 167
Normal, foot, 274; heart, 221; kidney, 269; liver, 231, 243;
    muscle, 299; pancreas, 277; sciatic nerve, 125
Northern fowl mite, 197
Nutritional deficiencies, 198-224

Oedma, lungs, sudden death syndrome, 233, 235; trachea,
    Newcastle disease, 104
Omphalitis, 22-27
Opisthotonos, encephalomalacia, 202
Orange-brown, mucus, small intestine, coccidiosis, 186
Ornithonyssus sylviarum, 197
Osteomyelitis, staphylococcal infection, 31-32
Osteopetrosis, 150
Ova, degenerate, 67
Ovary, degenerate ova, 67; moult, 303
Oviduct, carcinoma, 158; cystic dilation, 305; leiomyoma, 161;
    prolapse, 307; salpingitis, 5, 8-10

Pale, heart, fatty liver kidney syndrome, 221; kidney, fatty liver
    kidney syndrome, 220; liver, fatty liver kidney syndrome,
    218; muscles, coccidiosis, 179
Pancreas, fibrosed, 277-279; lymphoid infiltration, 117-118;
    normal, 277
Paralysis, toes, 199; transient, 138-139
Parasitic diseases, 176-197
Parathyroid, enlargement, rickets, 212
Paresis, Marek's disease, 124
Pasteurella multocida infection, 13-21
Periacinar fatty change, hepatocytes, congestive heart failure,
    246
Pericarditis, Coli septicaemia, 1, 6
Perihepatitis, Coli septicaemia, 1
Peripheral nerve, lymphocytes and plasma cells, 128
Peritonitis, Coli bacillosis, 7; fowl cholera, 17
Perivascular cuffing, Marek's disease, 137, 139; Newcastle
    disease, 106
Persistent right oviduct, 305
Pharynx, pox lesions, 96
'Pink disease', 217
Plantar pododermatitis, 301
Pneumonia, aspergillosis, 164; mycoplasmosis, 70-71;

Newcastle disease, 102; fowl cholera, 19-21
Pododermatitis, plantar, 302
Poor thriving, 309-311
Pox, fowl, 96-97
Prolapse, oviduct, 307
Protrusion, cloaca, sudden death syndrome, 236
Proventriculus, haemorrhages, 103; lymphoid infiltration, 119;
    swelling, 282
Pseudo-hyphae, candidiasis, 174-175
Pseudomonas aeruginosa infection, 153
Pyknosis, Marek's disease, 136

Red, liver, erythroid leukosis, 149; congestive heart failure,
    241
Red mite, 196
Renal failure, 263-275
Reovirus infection, 28, 120-123
Reticulo-endotheliosis virus-induced tumours, 157
Reticulolysis, fatty liver haemorrhagic syndrome, 230
Riboflavin deficiency, 198-201
Ribs, distorted, 213-214; fractured, 215; tumours, 147; rickety
    rosary, 207
Rickets, 267-212; stunting, 284
Roughened mucosa, small intestine, 187
Round heart disease, 247-248
Rounded cytoplasmic bodies, liver, cardiohepatic syndrome,
    239-240
Ruptured, gastrocnemius tendon, 120, 292; liver, fatty liver
    haemorrhagic syndrome, 225-226, 229; spleen, Marek's
    disease, 129

Salmonella gallinarum infection, 63-64
Salmonella pullorum infection, 65-67
Salmonella typhimurium infection, 59-62
Salmonellosis, 59-67
Salpingitis, Colibacillosis, 5, 8-10
Scabbed head, erysipelas, 48
Scaly leg, 194
Schwann cell proliferation, riboflavin deficiency, 200
Sciatic nerve, discoloured, 200; normal, 125; Schwann cell
    proliferation, 201
Septicaemia, coli, see Coli septicaemia
Shell, egg, abnormal, 111, 113
Sinuses, infraorbital, *M. gallisepticum*, 68-69
Skin, squamous cell carcinoma, 162-163; tumour, 132; wet,
    inflamed, 43-44
Small, liver, congestive heart failure, 242-243
Small intestine, dark contents, 222; distended, 183, 190;
    necrosis, 36-40, 189; orange-brown mucus, 186; pale and
    distended, 177; parasitism of epithelium, 188; roughened
    mucosa, 187
Spinal cord, compression, 289-291; encephalomyelitis, 115
Spleen, congestion, 6, 64; eosinophilic coagulum, 3;
    intranuclear inclusions, 95; tumours, 129, 153
Spondylolisthesis, 288-291
Squamous cell carcinoma, 162-163
Staphylococcal infection, 28-35, 45, 76
Staphylococcus aureus infection, 28-35
Sternum, bursitis, 72; tumour, 147; twisted, 213
Streptococcal infection, 35
Stunting syndrome, 276-283
Sudden death syndrome, 232-235, 236-237
Swollen, see Hypertrophy
Synovial membrane, inflamed, 77